Praise for Recognizing and Surviving Heart Attacks and Strokes

"The last thirty years have witnessed a therapeutic revolution in the management of acute myocardial infarction, which affects almost one million Americans per year. The ability to dissolve clots in the coronary arteries either with drugs or mechanically using transcatheter techniques has provided us with the ability to interrupt what was considered an inevitable process leading to irreversible loss of heart muscle. Many of the medical questions have been answered, and at the start of the twenty-first century it is not so much 'the nature of the treatment but the efficacy of its delivery' which determines outcome. The concept of 'time is muscle' holds true today, and time to treatment is a crucial determinant of success, which often means a return to a completely normal life.

The major source of treatment delays is patient-related. The more the patient understands the early warning signs of heart attack and how to respond to these and what treatments are available, the greater will be the beneficial impact of treatment on the community as a whole.

Doctor Turner is a pioneer in the field, and this important book reflects his passion and commitment to the field, a commitment that spans almost fifty years of public education, innovation, and implementation, in his native Missouri, nationally and internationally. The information he provides is vital but also should be considered as a source of encouragement since all of it points in a positive direction. The care of this deadly disease involves a partnership among physicians, all healthcare providers, and the patient. This book makes an important contribution to the field."

—Bernard J. Gersh, M.B.Ch.B., D.Phil., Cardiovascular Diseases, Mayo Clinic, Rochester, Minnesota

"This book presents to the general public an unequaled overview of how to reduce the nation's greatest health problem, the enormous death rate from heart attacks and strokes, the majority of which occur outside the hospital before patients arrive for the wonderful means of treatment now available in the hospital. Dr. Turner's unsurpassed approach, derived from nearly five decades of caring for thousands of patients in his cardiology practice encompassing the broad rural/urban Ozarks region of Southwest Missouri, is presented in this book in a highly readable fashion and is immediately useful to readers. During this period of public education concerning diseases of the heart and circulation he introduced the Early Warning Signs of a Heart Attack, adopted by the American Heart Association. His experience as a cardiologist and educator enabled him to also devise a very successful program of heart disease and stroke prevention. Dr. Turner's teachings have been very popular with people at all levels from elementary classrooms through adulthood."

—Valentin Fuster, M.D., Ph.D., Professor of Medicine–Cardiology, Mount Sinai School of Medicine, New York, New York

"The American public needs to be fully cognizant that receiving lifesaving treatment depends on one's recognizing and responding quickly to the early warning signs. . . . Dr. Turner's message is a truly lifesaving one."

—Hugh E. Stephenson, Jr., M.D., Growdon Distinguished Professor of Surgery Emeritus, University of Missouri–Columbia

"Anyone interested in understanding the signs and symptoms of heart disease as well as those wanting to know what they can do to avoid it will find this book not only interesting but also inspiring. Dr. Turner should be commended for passing on a half-century of clinical acumen."

—Thomas N. Levin, M.D., Director, Coronary Care Unit, Advocate Christ Medical Center, Oak Lawn, Illinois

Recognizing and Surviving Heart Attacks and Strokes

Recognizing and Surviving Heart Attacks and Strokes

Lifesaving Advice You Need Now

Glenn O. Turner, M.D.,
of the Groundbreaking Missouri Heart Program

With Mark Bruce Rosin

Illustrations by Tim Bade

University of Missouri Press   Columbia and London

University of Missouri Press, Columbia, Missouri 65201
Printed and bound in the United States of America

(cloth) 5 4 3 2 1 12 11 10 09 08
(paper) 5 4 3 2 1 12 11 10 09 08

Library of Congress Cataloging-in-Publication Data

Turner, Glenn O.
Recognizing and surviving heart attacks and strokes : lifesaving advice you need now / by Glenn O. Turner with Mark Bruce Rosin; illustrations by Tim Bade.
p. cm.
Includes bibliographical references and index.
Summary: "Drawing on fifty years of patient care and information from the Missouri Heart Program, Turner explains how to recognize all of the early warning signs of heart attacks and strokes - including little-known signs - and how important it is to seek immediate treatment to save lives and prevent damage to the heart"—Provided by publisher.
ISBN 978–0-8262–1788-2 (hardcover alk. paper) — ISBN 978–0-8262–1794-3 (pbk. alk. paper)
1. Myocardial infarction—Popular works. 2. Coronary heart disease—Popular works. 3. Cerebrovascular disease—Popular works. I. Rosin, Mark Bruce. II. Title.
RC685.I6T87 2008
616.1'237—dc22 2007052494

♾ This paper meets the requirements of the American National Standard for Permanence of Paper for Printed Library Materials, Z39.48, 1984.

Designer: Jennifer Cropp
Typesetter: BookComp, Inc.
Printer and Binder: Thomson-Shore, Inc.
Typefaces: Eplica and Palatino

The University of Missouri Press offers its grateful acknowledgment to The Missouri Southern Foundation for a generous contribution in support of the publication of this book.

This book is dedicated to my dear wife, Frances, for whose wisdom, strength, and loving support I am eternally grateful. Being the spouse of a doctor is challenging, and Frances has handled the heavy demands of my twelve- to sixteen-hour workdays with the constant grace and love that make her so special not only to me but to family, friends, and patients as well.

This book is also dedicated to John Q. Hammons, my friend and patient for almost fifty years. By responding promptly to the early warning signs of a heart attack, John enabled me to treat him within thirty minutes of the onset of symptoms, and the success of that treatment strengthened my early conviction that my life's work was to educate others in learning these symptoms. This book grew out of that commitment, and it could not have been written without his generous contributions to the advancement of heart attack research, treatment, and public education.

I have deep gratitude for Sharan Chittenden who converted my thousands of handwritten pages into the content of this book.

Contents

Preface

This book has grown out of my five decades of work as a cardiologist and as a heart-care public educator in Missouri. So it could be said that the book, like me, is Missouri born and bred.

A few biographical facts: I was born in Ozark, Missouri, went to college at Missouri State University in Springfield and to medical school at the University of Missouri Medical School and Washington University School of Medicine in St. Louis, and did my residency at Washington University's Barnes Hospital before setting up my practice in Springfield, where I was on staff at St. John's Hospital for forty-seven years. At various times, I served as St. John's chief of staff, chairman of the cardiovascular care committee, director of the comprehensive cardiovascular care unit (CVCU) project, and director of planning of the Hammons Heart Institute.

This book is the product of my application in the rural and urban regions of Southwest Missouri, with a population of one million (commonly known as the Ozarks), of new ideas in the diagnosis, treatment, and prevention of heart and blood-vessel disease, including stroke. As I discuss in greater detail later, on coming to Springfield to practice cardiology in 1947 I was appalled to observe the high death rate from cardiovascular disease. The majority of these deaths resulted from heart attacks, most of which occurred outside the hospital.

In that period, our knowledge about the nature of heart disease and how to treat it was very limited, so we had little to offer even to those who did reach the hospital. But breakthroughs soon began to appear. The first was Dr. Irving Wright's introduction in 1948 of anticoagulant treatment of heart attack patients in the hospital. Anticoagulants are medications that stop blood from clotting, and their administration interrupts the clotting that causes a heart attack during the attack. My associate and I seized upon this for all our heart attack patients and extended it to long-term treatment after discharge to prevent recurrence. This outpatient treatment was soon applied to patients with irregular heart rhythms (atrial fibrillation; see Chapter 19), blood clots in the legs (thrombophlebitis), and some with strokes.

The problem was we had no means of informing the general public about these advances so they could present themselves for treatment. The answer came in 1949 when the American Heart Association (AHA) converted from a private academic society to a public organization with the purpose of raising funds for heart disease research. When the Missouri Heart Association was formed soon after, my background in public speaking in college came in handy because it equipped me to become an active fund-raiser, giving many scores of public addresses throughout southwestern Missouri and northern Arkansas.

Each meeting hall was a classroom in which I taught the public about heart disease. By far the most popular topic was my description of heart attack symptoms and the need to get attention—and anticoagulant treatment—immediately. I called these symptoms the "early warning signs of a heart attack."

As a result of my extensive campaign to educate people about the early warning signs of a heart attack, admissions of heart attack and other heart disease patients to St. John's Hospital increased sharply. In these early postwar years, there was a severe shortage of community physicians, and I became the long-term personal physician of more than a thousand patients at any given time.

At St. John's, we were in the forefront of utilizing each new breakthrough in heart attack treatment, and at times we initiated breakthroughs ourselves. The increase in heart patient admissions to St. John's led, in 1960, to the nation's first cardiovascular care unit, a forty-two-bed admission-to-discharge unit that included a seven-bed intensive-care section. This was the advent of a major advance in heart care, the "grouping concept." It brought together for the first time all high-risk heart patients and the equipment and nursing staff for immediate recognition and treatment of otherwise fatal emergencies before the doctor could get there. In just one year, this system reduced heart attack deaths in my practice alone from 23 percent to 16 percent.

It was in 1960 that I was able to interrupt a heart attack during the first thirty minutes of symptoms by injection of heparin (an anticoagulant) in Springfield-based hotel builder John Q. Hammons, at age forty, as a result of his having learned the early warning signs. Hammons, now eighty-eight, has received continuous warfarin anticoagulant treatment since and remains extremely active, having recently been named "corporate hotelier of the world" by *Hotels* magazine.

The year 1960 was also when the Cleveland Clinic's Mason Sones introduced coronary angiography, a technique for examining the blockage in arteries that we immediately made available to our Missouri patients. Increasing demand for space for heart patients at St. John's led to the opening of a new ninety-bed CVCU in 1970, with an environment designed to ease psychological stress. This innovation was called the "modern motel concept" of heart care–facility design and borrowed comfort features from hotel design. A cardiac catheterization laboratory and a heart surgery section were included. The first coronary bypass surgery was done at St. John's in 1972, among the first applications of this surgery outside university and major metropolitan centers.

With more hospital space available in the CVCU, I decided to conduct a multimedia public and professional educational program on the early warning signs of a heart attack to hasten patient hospital arrival and increase the number of admissions. Funding was denied by all national sources for fear of overloading hospitals with false alarms and possibly actually causing heart attacks by describing frightening symptoms, but the Missouri Heart Association granted the necessary funds.

The Missouri Early Warning Signs Public Education Program was launched in July 1971. Its results, described more fully later in the book, were startling in their success: the median time for patients to start to the hospital after the onset of symptoms was cut nearly in half. The effectiveness of the Missouri program made it the subject of national and international media coverage, and to date it is the only program in the United States to successfully hasten patient arrival for heart attack treatment. The American Heart Association was extremely impressed with the results, and its president, Paul Yu, sent accolades, as did other AHA executives Fred Arkus and Keith Thwaites. One of the primary reasons for this book is to make all the vital information in the program available to a national readership for the first time.

The Missouri program continued in southwestern Missouri throughout the 1970s and, in the 1980s, was succeeded by television and radio spots featuring the Claymation character "Heart Doctor."

These spots were financed by a grant of one hundred thousand dollars from Mr. Hammons. During that decade, he also provided the one million–dollar Hammons Lifeline helicopter dedicated to heart patient transport, and he financed the multimillion-dollar Hammons Heart Institute to support regional heart care. In the 1990s the Turner Heart Foundation was established to conduct a third-generation early-warning-signs program.

The Turner Foundation's predominant focus was providing illustrated articles for community newspapers, showing the early warning signs and urging patients to promptly call their doctors or immediately get to the nearest emergency room if heart attack or stroke symptoms appeared. Comprehensive information on the prevention of heart attacks and strokes was also given. There were also major television presentations, publications in the Missouri Southern State University magazine, and many addresses to the general public and to student groups starting at the elementary school level. Three years in a row the Turner Heart Foundation's early-warning-signs presentation was named the favorite of Asian exchange-student groups, and I received an invitation to lecture in China.

Forty of the fifty regional local newspapers accepted the foundation's articles. By the time forty-three columns had been published, the National Newspaper Association urged me to syndicate the articles nationally, but I believed a book would be preferable so that it could be kept on hand as a ready reference. That is the background of this book. It is based on my work as a cardiologist and public educator in heart attack and stroke early recognition and treatment. It is also based on research.

Missouri is famous for being the "Show Me State." As a Missourian, this has long been my motto. Don't just tell me something is true; prove it to me. In writing this book, I have examined the research—the latest data about heart attack and stroke treatment and prevention—and I am presenting these findings here. Thus, along with my firsthand experience as a cardiologist and personal physician, I am incorporating research to help you learn about the early recognition, treatment, and prevention of heart attacks and strokes.

Recognizing and Surviving Heart Attacks and Strokes

Introduction

Why This Book?

One of the greatest medical problems facing our country today is the occurrence of needless early deaths from heart attacks and strokes. This book will teach you to recognize the key early symptoms of heart attacks and strokes in order to get the quickest possible treatment. It will teach you about the best treatments available, what makes one treatment better than another, and what you can do to prevent initial and recurrent episodes of heart attacks and strokes. I guarantee this book will save the lives and reduce the disability of countless of its readers.

Of the more than one million heart attacks in the United States each year, nearly half result in death in the acute (early) stages.[1] It is difficult to comprehend the magnitude of this problem, but you can get some idea of it by realizing that coronary heart disease deaths in the United States annually, most from heart attacks,[2] exceed the total battle deaths of U.S. servicemen and -women in all the wars of the twentieth century, from World War I through the Gulf War.[3] The great majority of these heart attack deaths occur before patients are admitted to the hospital. If you have a heart attack, as matters now stand, your chance of dying approaches 50 percent. But this need not be so!

The reason so many people do not reach the hospital in time is that they fail to recognize the early warning signs of a heart attack and therefore do not respond soon enough to avail themselves of lifesaving treatment. On the other hand, when you learn these early warning signs and how to respond to them, in most cases you can reach the hospital in time to save your life and, in many cases, prevent disability.

Nationally, it takes the average patient 2.7 hours (that is, 2 hours, 42 minutes) after the onset of symptoms to arrive at the hospital.[4] By this time, the majority of heart attack deaths have already occurred. So at present, U.S. hospitals are treating only those who survive this deadly period of the illness. This means that there is still only a very limited reduction of death and disability risk from the early phase of the heart attack. Even for those who survive this period, irreversible damage to the heart is usually complete by 3 hours after symptoms begin, limiting the benefits of treatment given after such a long lapse, since heart muscle cannot be regenerated.

This is notwithstanding the great advances in treatment that are available if used in time. Clearly, the vital words are *in time*. The most effective treatment occurs during the first 60 minutes of symptoms, known as the "golden hour." Even up to 3 hours after the onset of symptoms, treatment can save valuable heart muscle and improve one's quality of life after recovery. Receiving this treatment depends on the patient recognizing and responding quickly to the early warning signs.

As you may know, virtually all heart attacks are caused by a narrowing of the arteries, known as atherosclerosis, a process I will explain in detail in Chapter 2. You may not know, however, that most strokes are also caused by atherosclerosis. For this reason, strokes, as well as heart attacks, have been the focus of my work as a cardiologist, and I will discuss them in this book, too.

Delayed recognition of stroke warnings also has costly consequences, since wonderful lifesaving and disability-reducing treatments are available if given during the first 3 hours of symptoms. As with heart attacks, I am going to teach you how to recognize the key early warning signs of a stroke so that, should these symptoms appear, you can get prompt treatment. And the guidelines I will present in Part V for the prevention of heart attacks will also help you to reduce the risk of a stroke.

That is the *why* of this book: to remove from your life the threat of needless death and disability from a heart attack and stroke.

I am writing on these vital subjects from the uncommon perspective of having spent more than fifty years as a cardiologist, starting in the U.S. Army during World War II. I have had firsthand experience with the many breakthroughs in heart care that occurred during this exciting period in the development of cardiology.

As an army doctor, I was among the first to diagnose heart attacks in young soldiers on the battlefield. After the war, when I returned to Springfield, Missouri, I served as the primary care cardiologist and personal physician to thousands of patients with heart and blood vessel disease in urban Springfield as well as in rural communities extending 125 miles to the east and 60 miles to the west. Because I was one of only two cardiologists in the region, my services were in great demand, and every year I had to buy a car to replace the one I had worn out traveling to patients. In this way, I gained experience with all aspects of cardiac care for patients living close to the major hospitals in Springfield as well as those living near smaller hospitals in rural areas.

I also devoted attention to the prevention of heart attacks and strokes by creating the Missouri Early Warning Signs Public Education Program, the only such program in the nation to bring about the earlier hospital arrival of heart attack patients. Everything I learned in conducting this program, and in the three and a half decades that followed, has informed the writing of this book, the first of its scope about heart attacks and strokes.

My commitment to teaching people what they could do to save their own lives grew out of my early experiences as a cardiologist in and around Springfield. Even after treating men with heart attacks amid the violence of war, it was shocking to me to come home and see that so many people died of heart attacks outside the hospital, many even before I reached their homes. At that time, I believed that most of my job as a cardiologist was signing death certificates. After leaving a heart attack victim's home, I sometimes wept not only to have seen a forty-year-old man who had died in his prime but also to have witnessed the indescribable grief of his wife and children.

After their husbands died, the widows became my patients, and as the years passed I saw that they, too, were subject to heart disease. This led me to be among the first to recognize the great frequency of heart attacks in women at later ages. All the while, I kept wondering if there was anything that could be done to help people get to the hospital more quickly. Was there nothing that I could do personally?

At that time, even when patients reached the hospital, treatment consisted only of morphine for pain relief and three to six weeks of absolute bed rest to allow the heart to heal. Fortunately, breakthroughs in cardiac care soon began to arrive, starting with Dr. Wright's introduction of anticoagulants to treat heart attack patients[5] and the exciting conversion of the American Heart Association into a public fund-raising organization.

As a fund-raiser for the new Missouri Affiliate of the AHA, I addressed countless community groups. I soon found that opening each talk with a brief summary of heart attack symptoms guaranteed audience attention. I also found that advising them to call their doctors or get to the hospital quickly if any of these symptoms appeared led to a steady flow of telephone calls to physicians and more hospital admissions for patients experiencing the early stages of heart attacks. This exciting experience was key to my future path as a cardiologist. It showed me that public education about heart attack symptoms and prompt response could work. Concurrently, although my primary focus was heart attacks, I became actively involved in stroke care, as it was clear that in so many cases the cause was the same as for heart attacks: narrowing of the arteries.

My public education outreach about early warning signs not only increased the number of heart attack patients coming to St. John's but also attracted additional physicians. Many of us were intensively involved in cardiac care, and under my direction we established the nation's first cardiovascular care unit. Recognizing the strong connection between patients who had heart attacks and many of those who had strokes, I included improved stroke care in this new facility as well.

At our first planning meeting for the CVCU, Dr. Cecil Auner observed, "It seems almost immoral to be spending all these millions on hospital facilities when most of the heart attack deaths are still occurring before the patient gets to the hospital." Auner's statement strengthened my resolve to create a comprehensive regionwide public education program on the early warning signs of heart attacks so that we could get more patients to the hospital sooner and save more lives.

The launch of the Missouri program (officially known as the Greene County Heart Association Early Warning Signs of Heart Attack Public and Professional Education Program) gave us the means not just to educate the public about the early warning signs and strengthen communication between physicians and patients but also to collect data that told us how well we were doing. As a result of this program, the time required for patients and their families to decide to start to the hospital after symptoms began was reduced from 4 hours to 2.2 hours.[6] Admissions of CVCU patients who suspected they were having heart attacks increased by 60 percent, the great majority of whom did prove to have actual or developing heart attacks.

In the past few decades, public awareness of heart attack symptoms has grown, beginning with the national media's coverage of our Missouri program. With the program's success, suddenly newspapers and magazines throughout the country were communicating vital information about early warning signs to their readers. When the *Reader's Digest* published an article about the Missouri program in its thirty-plus worldwide editions, it received letter after letter from readers saying their lives had been saved by the information.

But despite our program's effectiveness, there has never been a national public education program about early warning signs. Statistics show that even today, too few people recognize the early signs of a heart attack or, if they do recognize them, fail to respond early enough. This is all the more sad because of the tremendous innovations in heart care that are now available. Similarly, there has never been a public education program about the early warning signs of a stroke.

Again, that is the *why* of this book: to help you avoid needless death and disability from a heart attack or stroke. This requires a fourfold approach: first, and by far the most important, learning the early warning signs of heart attacks and strokes; second, greatly enhancing your knowledge and judgment about the best way to respond to these symptoms should they occur; third, learning what treatments are available once you reach the hospital and how, in conjunction with your physician, to exercise your extremely important personal prerogatives in choosing the type and place of treatment—knowledge that will help you navigate your way through today's often confusing medical world and get the best care possible; and fourth, learning how you can reduce the risk of heart attacks and strokes through diet and exercise.

You will find all of this vital information in *Recognizing and Surviving Heart Attacks and Strokes: Lifesaving Advice You Need Now.* When we launched our public education work in Missouri, one of my media advisers told me, "Dr. Turner, you need to sell this information, saying it and saying it again till people get it!" I took his advice, and he proved right. So I am going to give you information on heart care and strokes as if I were selling you a service. I am going to repeat the essential lifesaving lessons you need to learn until they become second nature to you. For some of you, learning this information may seem scary. Medical knowledge, particularly about disease, or even disease prevention, is something many people prefer to avoid for fear that it will make them focus on the possibility of illness. But as you will see, knowing the symptoms of heart attacks and strokes means early recognition, early recognition gives you the ability to respond promptly, responding promptly gives you the ability to get early treatment, and early treatment can save your life!

Part I

How to Recognize and Respond to the Early Warning Signs of a Heart Attack

CHAPTER 1

Your Heart

What It Is and How It Functions

The more you learn about your heart, I am sure the more you will agree how incredible it is. Here are the basic facts: Your heart weighs about twelve ounces if you are a man and about eight ounces if you are a woman (fig. 1.1). It consists of an interweaving of long muscle fibers. When these fibers contract and shorten, the heart contracts, expelling blood from its chambers to start its circulation throughout the body. The bulk of this round muscular pump is in the midline of your chest (fig. 1.2), between your right and left lungs. It extends downward and somewhat to the left, the tip (or apex) being behind your left breast nipple. Many people believe that the heart is in the left side of the chest, but, in fact, except for its apex or tip, it is in the middle.

The Structure of the Heart

The Heart Chambers

The heart has four chambers (fig. 1.3). The chambers on top are called atria. They have far thinner walls than the chambers on the bottom, which are called ventricles. The reason they have thinner

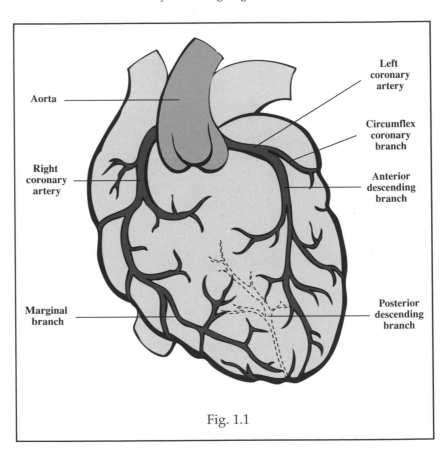

Aorta
Left coronary artery
Circumflex coronary branch
Right coronary artery
Anterior descending branch
Marginal branch
Posterior descending branch

Fig. 1.1

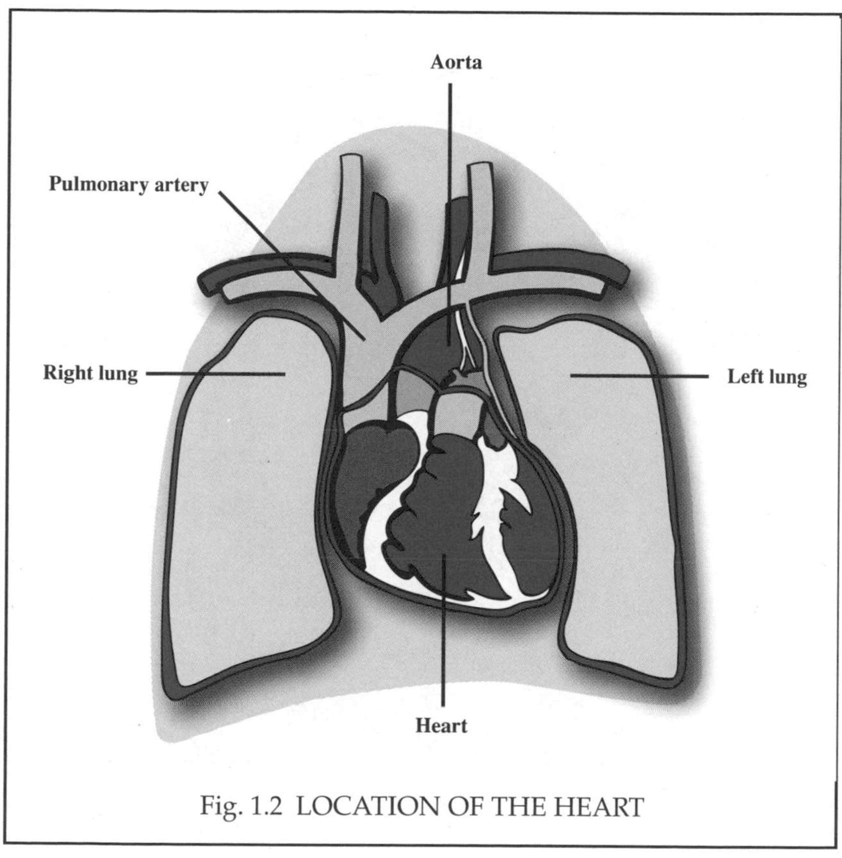

Fig. 1.2 LOCATION OF THE HEART

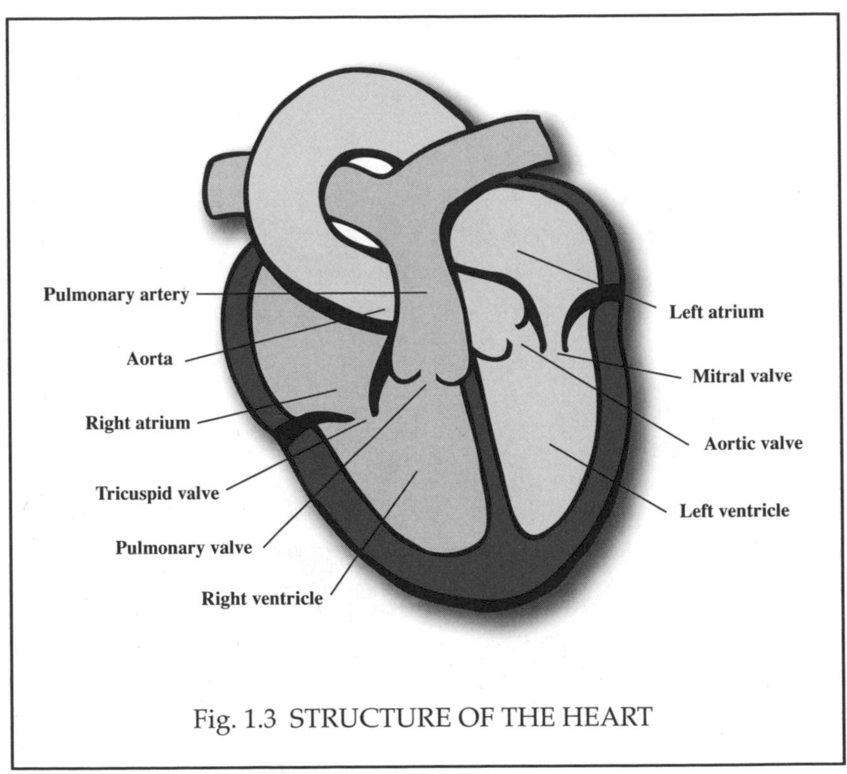

Fig. 1.3 STRUCTURE OF THE HEART

walls is that the right and left atria are primarily collecting chambers, and although they pump the blood into the ventricles, they do so at a lower pressure than the pressure of the pumping action of the ventricles that pump blood into the body.

The right atrium receives used blood from the body, via your veins, and then, with its low-pressure pumping action, empties it into the right ventricle. The more thickly walled right ventricle forces the blood through the pulmonary arteries into the lungs to be replenished with oxygen and to discard carbon dioxide, the by-product of the used oxygen. The rejuvenated blood then passes into the left atrium. With low pressure, this blood is passed into the left ventricle, the thick-walled high-pressure pump that delivers fresh blood throughout the body via the extensive peripheral artery system.

The Heart Valves

The heart has four valves. These flaps, or cusps, are of very thin, extremely tough tissue. They open widely and close snugly. The tricuspid is situated between the right atrium and right ventricle, and the mitral is between the left atrium and left ventricle. Two additional valves separate the ventricles from the arteries to which they deliver blood. The pulmonary valve is between the right ventricle and the pulmonary artery. The aortic valve separates the left ventricle and the aorta, the largest artery in the body.

The Aorta

Our main artery, with a diameter of about an inch, originates at the top of the heart (see figs. 1.1–1.3) and delivers fresh blood throughout the body. The first branches are the coronary arteries, which carry blood back to the heart muscle. Arising from the aorta above the coronary arteries are the carotid arteries, which carry blood to the brain and the rest of the head (see Chapter 22). Next are branches to the arms, abdominal organs, kidneys, and legs. The wall of the aorta has three layers and is highly expansible.

The Coronary Arteries

The two matchstick-size coronary arteries are the fuel lines to our heart. They branch off the aorta just above the aortic valve, and are known simply as the left coronary artery and right coronary artery.

The left coronary artery divides soon after it leaves the aorta, forming the anterior descending branch, which goes down the front center of your heart, and the left circumflex branch, which extends around the left side of your heart to the back of the heart. The right coronary artery extends around the right side of your heart to the back of the heart. There, along with the left circumflex artery, it supplies blood to the back of your heart.

Thus, there are three primary arterial channels supplying blood to your heart: the anterior descending, the left circumflex, and the right coronary artery. They branch progressively into a myriad of microscopic channels that deliver nutrients directly to the individual heart muscle cells.

Like the aorta, these three main artery channels and their major branches have walls of three layers and expand with each heartbeat and then contract. The innermost layer is the extremely thin lining known as the intima. The second layer is the media, which makes up most of the bulk of the normal artery and is highly elastic. The outermost layer is the rather thin, tough tissue encasement called the adventitia.

The Coronary Veins

The thin-walled coronary veins run alongside the coronary arteries and carry used blood back from the heart muscle to be rejuvenated by the lungs, where they also dispose of waste products (such as carbon dioxide). After rejuvenation and waste elimination, the blood then returns to the left ventricle, where it is then pumped throughout the body.

The Vena Cava

The vena cava is the large vein that lies alongside the aorta and collects used blood from veins throughout the body, delivering it to the right atrium for replenishment.

The Heart's Electrical System

We have an amazing electrical system in our hearts. The sinoatrial (SA) node is a tiny nodule of tissue on top of the atria (the upper chambers of the heart) with its own self-contained electricity generator that initiates the rhythmic heartbeat. Connected to the SA node from above are "sympathetic" and "parasympathetic" nerves, which speed up or slow down the heart rate.

Lying between the atria and ventricles is the atrioventricular (AV) node. It passes the SA signals on to the ventricles. This sends electricity down through a special nerve known as the "Bundle of His" (named after Swiss internist, biochemist, and cardiologist Wilhelm His Jr., who discovered it). The Bundle of His divides into left and right bundle branches, which distribute electrical signals into the ventricles to cause them to contract at a certain pace.

The Pericardium

The pericardium is a very thin, snugly fitting pouch containing the heart, with internal lubricants to reduce friction as the heart pumps.

How the Heart Functions

The SA node establishes the rhythm of the heart. During exercise, excitement, or blood loss, the sympathetic nerves speed up the heart. During sleep, the parasympathetic nerves slow it down. The SA node's electrical signal causes the atria to contract, emptying their contents into the ventricles. During a period of about one-sixth of a second, the signal passes through the walls of the atria to the AV node. This signals the ventricles to contract. The simultaneous contraction of the ventricles causes an ejection of the blood they contain into the aorta and pulmonary artery, which requires about one-twelfth of a second. This leaves about eleven-twelfths of a second for the ventricles to rest before the next beat.

This is how a normal heart survives for a lifetime. Blood passes through the aorta at a speed of about fifty miles an hour. To achieve this rate of flow, the heart generates pressure sufficient to pump a column of water six feet upward. This pressure is recorded in millimeters of mercury. Normal is generally considered to be 120/80 (see Chapter 39 on blood pressure). The veins return blood at a slower rate and under less pressure. When we are resting, the heart normally beats sixty to ninety times per minute, but that rate may double during exercise. These heart rates cause the pumping of a remarkable quantity of blood every minute. Each drop of blood makes a complete round-trip through the system of arteries and veins every twenty seconds, or three round-trips per minute.

Our hearts are precious. We must do our best to make them last as long as possible.

CHAPTER 2

What Is a Heart Attack?

Technically known as an acute myocardial infarction, or AMI, a heart attack is the most challenging and formidable of the important disorders of the heart and circulatory system. Other heart problems include congestive heart failure, heart rhythm disturbances, diseases of the valves, aortic aneurysm, and congenital heart anomalies. I am focusing exclusively on heart attacks and strokes.

A heart attack consists of the obstruction of blood flow through a coronary artery, which deprives heart muscle downstream of oxygen and other nutrients, causing that portion of the heart wall to die (fig. 2.1). The artery blockage may be in one of the three main channels of the coronary arteries or in one of their branches, and thus may occur in the front, right or left side, or back of the heart.

The size of the vessel that is blocked, or occluded, determines the extent of heart muscle damage. A heart attack may be mild, moderate, or severe. The immediate diagnosis is by electrocardiogram (ECG), which discloses the shortage of blood supply to the heart muscle due to the artery blockage. When the death of heart muscle involves the total thickness of the ventricle wall, it shows up in ECG changes that identify it as a "Q Wave" or "ST Segment Elevation Infarction." When only partial thickness of the wall is deprived of blood, it is known as a "Non–Q Wave Infarction." ECG testing reveals the location and physical extent of heart muscle damage. Blood tests reveal the severity of heart muscle damage. In emergency rooms (ERs), the ECG can be done in less than eight minutes after arrival and blood tests soon after.

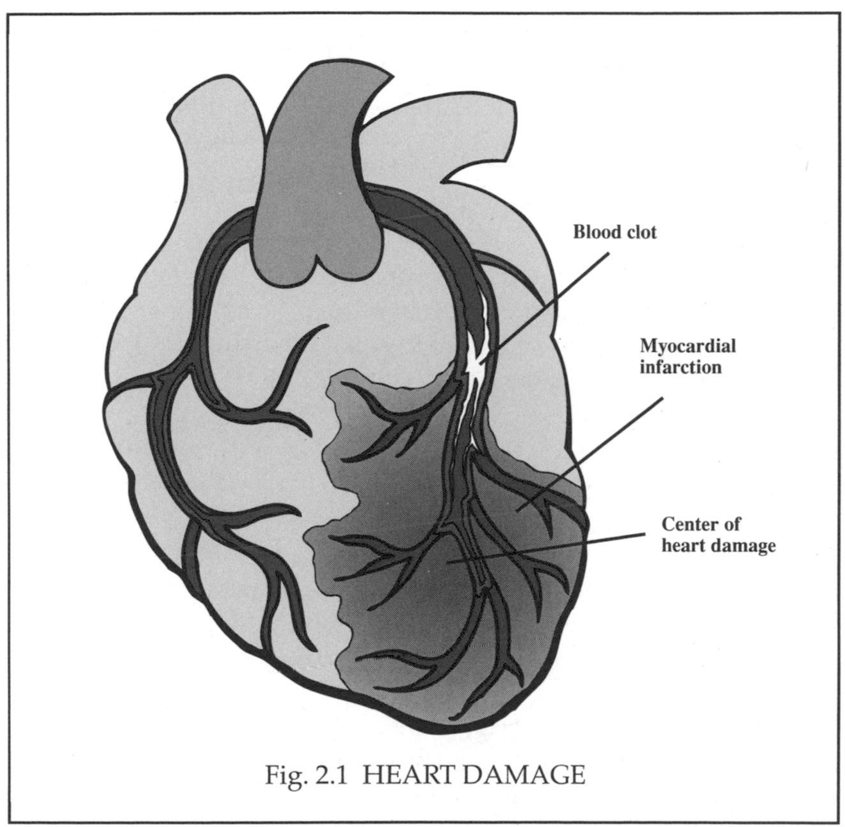

Fig. 2.1 HEART DAMAGE

The most serious heart attacks are those caused by obstruction of the left coronary artery before it branches, because that deprives the front, left side, and part of the back of the heart of blood. Next in severity is blockage of the anterior descending artery, because it deprives the entire front of the heart of blood (see fig 2.1). It is generally agreed that the death of heart muscle is complete after being deprived of blood for three hours after artery obstruction. Once the death of blood-deprived heart muscle has occurred, life of that muscle cannot be restored, although research is going on in the attempt to bring that about.

Do not be confused: *Even when heart muscle in a particular part of the heart has died, it does not mean that a person will necessarily die.* With proper treatment, people can survive for decades with loss of as much as 40 percent of their heart. But it is not necessary for any heart muscle to die just because an artery becomes obstructed by a blood clot, the most common reason for most blockages. This is why knowing and responding quickly to the early warning signs is so important.

In the 1970s, researchers discovered effective agents to dissolve blood clots in the coronary arteries. The first successful treatment was in 1979 by Dr. Peter Rentrop.[1] This process of dissolving blood clots is called thrombolysis. Soon after the introduction of thrombolysis to dissolve the clots that cause most heart attacks, studies found that giving this treatment during the first sixty minutes of symptoms cut deaths in half and giving it before the end of the third hour of symptoms cut deaths by 25 percent.[2] A later U.S. study showed that the death rate in patients treated with thrombolysis during the first seventy minutes of symptoms was 1.2 percent, compared with 8.7 percent in those treated later.[3] One recent study showed that, among patients who received thrombolysis during the first sixty minutes of symptoms, 30 percent sustained no heart damage at all.[4] Because of the benefit provided by early treatment, shortly after the introduction of thrombolysis, I termed the first sixty minutes the "golden hour," a phrase that was soon widely adopted by members of the medical profession.

Most people have heard about blood clots causing heart attacks, and most know that usually cholesterol, a lipid (or fat) that is a normal component of the blood, is also associated with heart attacks, but few understand how these factors actually contribute to an attack.

The process leading to an obstruction in the coronary artery that will cause a heart attack is the depositing of low-density lipoprotein cholesterol, widely known as LDL, or "bad," cholesterol in the artery wall. (See Chapters 11, 12, and 13 for more details about cholesterol and other blood lipids.) These LDL deposits—known as plaques—are underneath the thin intima lining of the artery and also extend into the middle layer of the artery, the media. Over the years, the plaques gradually increase in thickness, as shown in fig. 2.2, and produce a condition known as atherosclerosis, or hardening of the arteries.

Until fairly recently, it was believed that heart attacks resulted from complete obstruction of the blood vessel by the atherosclerotic plaque. It was also believed that blood clots found there were formed after cholesterol had completely closed the artery. It was recognized that the discomfort on exertion known as angina (see Chapter 4) is

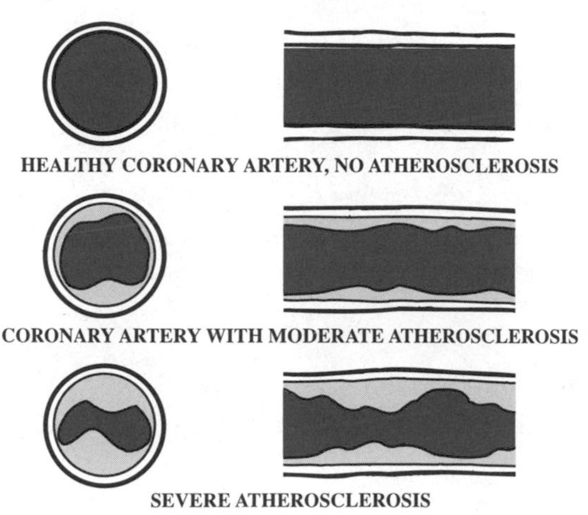

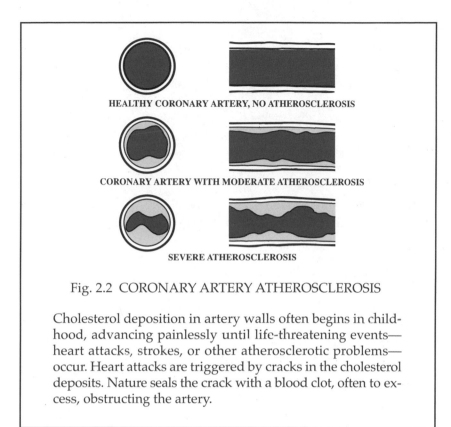

Fig. 2.2 CORONARY ARTERY ATHEROSCLEROSIS

Cholesterol deposition in artery walls often begins in childhood, advancing painlessly until life-threatening events—heart attacks, strokes, or other atherosclerotic problems—occur. Heart attacks are triggered by cracks in the cholesterol deposits. Nature seals the crack with a blood clot, often to excess, obstructing the artery.

due to marked narrowing of the artery by cholesterol, preventing adequate blood flow through the artery during exertion. Surprisingly, however, it was discovered that most heart attacks occur during the early stages of cholesterol depositing, when the plaques are thin. The expanding of the artery with each heartbeat causes cracks in the covering of the plaques. This injury to the artery then leads to the normal healing process of nature, sealing the crack with a blood clot. It is thought that in most cases this sealing action is correct and not harmful, but in some cases the clot formation is excessive, and the clot becomes large enough to partly or completely obstruct the artery, interfering with blood flow to heart muscle downstream. If the blockage is incomplete, heart attack symptoms may at first be very mild or even intermittent, worsening as the obstruction increases or becomes complete (fig. 2.3).

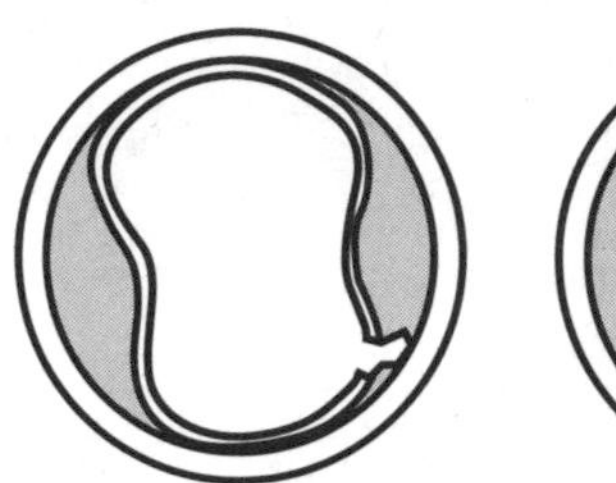

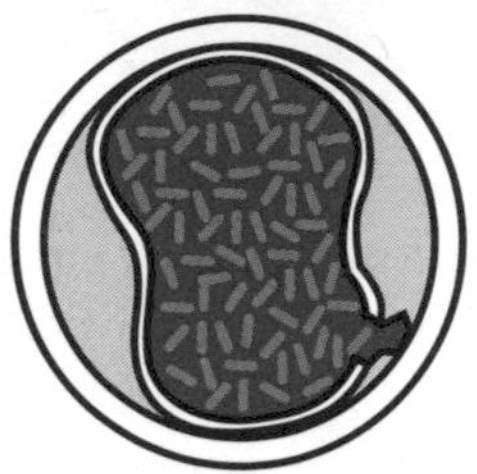

Fig. 2.3

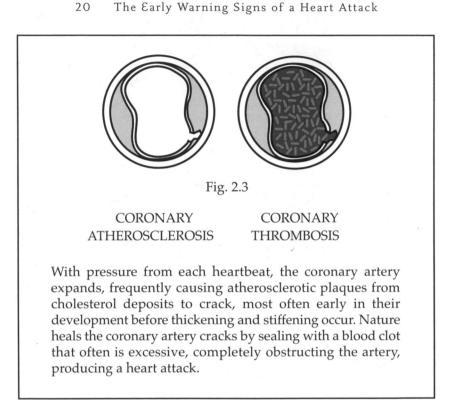

CORONARY ATHEROSCLEROSIS

CORONARY THROMBOSIS

With pressure from each heartbeat, the coronary artery expands, frequently causing atherosclerotic plaques from cholesterol deposits to crack, most often early in their development before thickening and stiffening occur. Nature heals the coronary artery cracks by sealing with a blood clot that often is excessive, completely obstructing the artery, producing a heart attack.

It is extremely important that you understand this process so that you can act quickly in the event of a heart attack. Time may elapse between an artery beginning to narrow, which results in mild or intermittent symptoms, and complete obstruction of the artery, which results in more severe symptoms and greater damage to the heart if flow is not restored. Therefore, there may be a period during which, if you are able to recognize and respond to the earliest symptoms, you may have sufficient time for treatment to interrupt the increasing clotting of blood before complete artery obstruction and severe consequences occur.

The lesser degrees of artery narrowing by blood clots are now widely known as acute coronary syndrome (ACS). My observation of this process in patients led me to come up with the saying, "Heart attacks don't just happen—they develop. Early attention may mean prevention of heart damage." Your knowledge of this process can save your life by helping you respond quickly to the early warning signs.

To summarize: Blockage of an artery—the most common cause of heart attacks—deprives a portion of the heart of blood. Unless the artery is reopened within three hours, the heart muscle downstream dies. Reopening the artery before three hours saves muscle, the amount depending on how soon blood flow is restored. How this is accomplished is described in Part II.

There are several possible consequences of a coronary artery becoming obstructed. First and most lethal is the heart rhythm disturbance known as ventricular fibrillation. When the normal once-a-second (or so) electrical heartbeat signal passes downward into the ventricular muscle and reaches an area of muscle with no blood supply, the rhythmic signal may be transformed, becoming completely disorganized. This disorganized signal spreads throughout the ventricle, converting the normally rhythmic heart into a writhing motion that pumps no blood (fig. 2.4). In this state, the heart has sometimes been described as resembling a writhing bag of worms. The chaotic rhythm can be stopped only by passing an electric current through the chest wall into the heart by a device known as a defibrillator.

Ventricular fibrillation causes virtually all the heart attack deaths that occur before hospital arrival. Most of these deaths occur during the first two hours of symptoms. To be effective in stopping ventricular fibrillation, electrical defibrillation must be carried out during the first several minutes after onset of the heart attack, unless a bystander applies chest compression to maintain blood flow until a defibrillator is available later. Only a small percentage of resuscitations outside the hospital are successful.

This is why early recognition of symptoms and early hospital arrival are the best means of improving survival from a heart attack. In the hospital, with continuous monitoring of the heart rhythm, an episode of ventricular fibrillation can be immediately stopped by defibrillation. Medication can usually prevent subsequent episodes.

The second most serious consequence of an artery becoming obstructed is that so much of the heart muscle is lost from the blockage that the remaining muscle cannot sustain the blood pressure necessary to maintain blood flow. This is known as cardiogenic shock. It requires urgent life support measures. If a smaller amount of heart muscle is lost, the blood pressure may be maintained, but flow may be impaired. One effect of this is the backup of blood in the lungs,

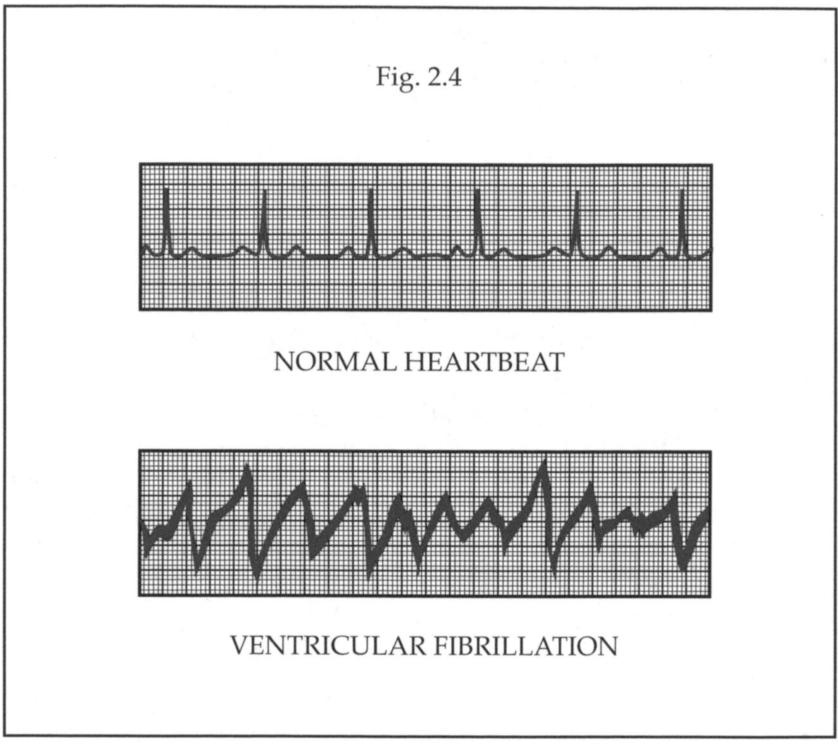

causing shortness of breath, a complication known as congestive heart failure. Congestive heart failure is one of the leading causes of hospitalization in the United States.

If blood flow is cut off to the main nerve channel carrying heartbeat signals down into the ventricle, a condition known as "heart block" occurs. A patient with heart block requires a pacemaker to stimulate the ventricles to beat rhythmically after the main electrical channel is cut off.

If blood flow is cut off in a branch of the main nerve channel but not in the primary channel, it is called right or left bundle-branch block. This condition is less serious. Treatment for it includes the implantation of special pacemakers that make the two sides of the heart beat equally.

A third possible consequence of coronary artery blockage is heart valve damage. When the heart valve leading to the left ventricle is severely impaired, surgical correction or valve replacement is necessary.

In a minority of people, muscular damage from a heart attack produces a softening of the left or right ventricle wall, which can then rupture. This can be repaired only through surgery.

In most cases, damage in the ventricles caused by arterial blockages does not create a rupture of the muscle. When no rupture occurs, healing of the damaged area of the heart wall is accomplished by the formation of scar tissue. This requires three to six weeks, and the process is similar to the healing of skin. If the damaged area is very broad, the heart wall becomes thinner. The thinner heart wall may then bulge outward, causing a protuberance known as ventricular aneurysm. When a ventricular aneurysm is large, it may require surgical removal.

Even when the damaged heart muscle is healed, it may distort the passage of heartbeat signals through that area, causing ventricular fibrillation or intolerable rapid heart action known as ventricular tachycardia. Since these possibly lethal heart rhythm disturbances occur without forewarning, prevention requires intensive long-term drug administration or the implantation of an automatic defibrillator. This latter treatment has proved to be more effective, and hundreds of thousands of people are successfully using it today.

Other less serious heart rhythm disturbances may occur after heart attacks caused by artery blockage and are usually manageable with medications.

With all of this in mind, you can see why early recognition, prompt treatment, and lifetime prevention measures can help to avoid dangerous complications and possibly avoid any damage at all.

CHAPTER 3

Heart Attack Early Warning Signs

Your Key to Survival

In the United States the average delay in reaching the hospital after the onset of heart attack symptoms is 2.7 hours. Clearly, with what you now know about damage done to the heart in three hours, you want to get to the hospital much sooner—preferably during the golden hour, that is, the first sixty minutes after the onset of symptoms.

The first step in getting to the hospital quickly is recognition of the early warning signs of a heart attack. Again, the key word is *early*—you don't want to wait for later signs, for symptoms that are intermittent to become persistent or to worsen. Once you know the early warning signs of a heart attack, you can make a judgment within one or two minutes after the appearance of symptoms.

The following information can save your life. Memorize it as you would memorize how to escape a hotel in case of fire. You don't want the emergency to occur, but it is necessary to know how to respond if it does. In the case of a heart attack, getting to the hospital in time is as crucial as getting penicillin or other antibiotics to stop a possibly lethal infection.

Since the heart is in the center of the front of the chest, the warning discomfort of a heart attack most frequently occurs in this area (fig. 3.1). The discomfort is usually a feeling of pressure, fullness, squeezing, aching, or burning. It may extend into one or both arms, the neck,

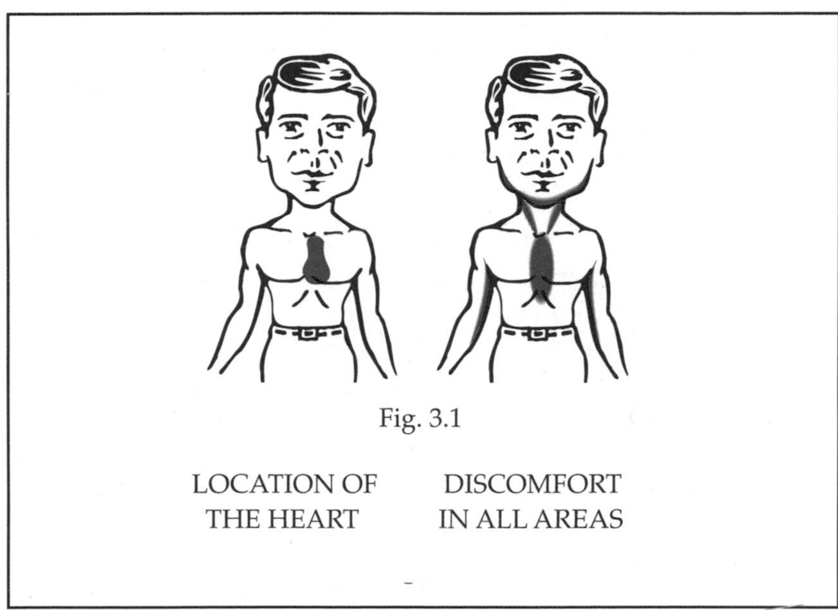

Fig. 3.1

LOCATION OF THE HEART — DISCOMFORT IN ALL AREAS

jaws, upper abdomen, or back. It can occur simultaneously in all of these areas, in any one area, or in combinations of areas. Discomfort can occur in one or both arms, in the neck or jaws, or in the upper abdomen without being in the chest at all.

Indeed, a study by the National Registry of Myocardial Infarction of 434,877 patients who sustained a heart attack showed that 33 percent—one-third—had no chest pain or chest discomfort. Thus, for many people, the prevailing notion that chest pain always accompanies heart attacks has caused serious delay in response to other symptoms they do not recognize and has caused even further delay in hospital arrival.

You can usually tell the difference between chest discomfort from a heart attack and harmless left chest-wall pain. Harmless left chest-wall pain is generally muscular pain. It may be a dull discomfort or a brief jabbing pain well to the left of the center of your chest, in the region of the left breast. Recognizing harmless left chest-wall pain can save you an urgent trip to the hospital (fig. 3.2). A call to your doctor can usually resolve this matter by telephone once you explain the symptoms in detail. All chest discomfort must be investigated, but examination of non–heart attack chest-wall pain can be done at a

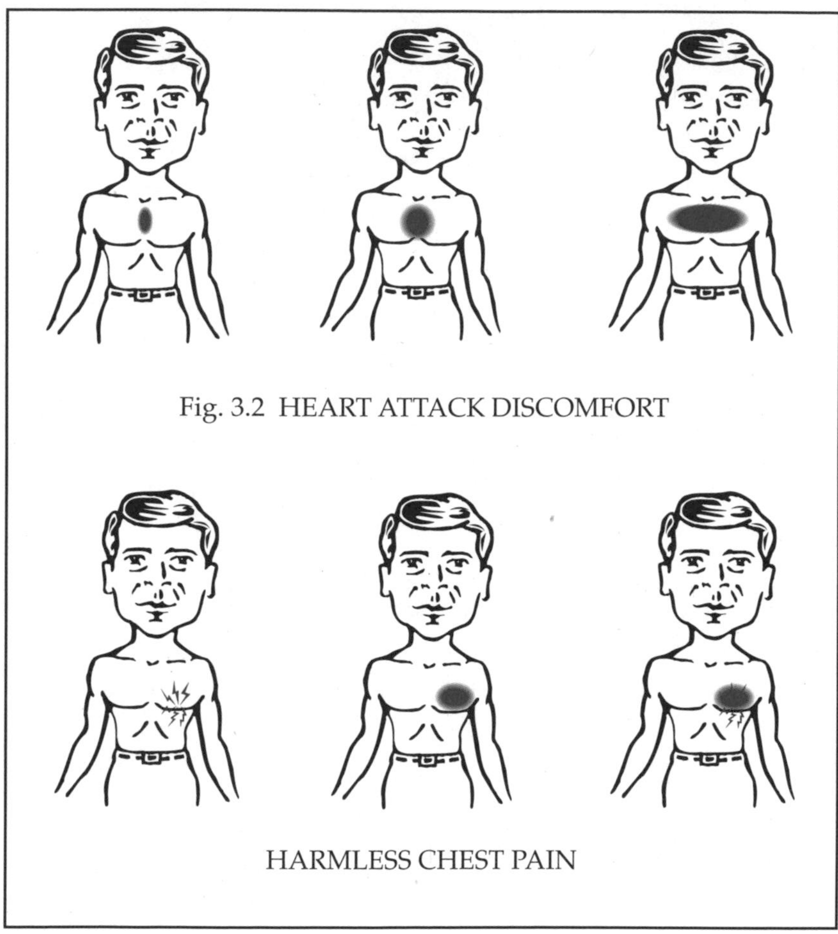

Fig. 3.2 HEART ATTACK DISCOMFORT

HARMLESS CHEST PAIN

later time more convenient for you. When uncertainty exists, it is best to go to the hospital.

These true-to-life illustrations will help you understand and memorize the possible patterns of heart attack discomfort and how they differ from harmless chest-wall discomfort. The information below about early warning signs can speed up your decision to seek help. *Remember, you are educating yourself to be aware of each symptom in itself; any of the symptoms can occur alone or in combination with any of the others, and no symptom is more important than another.* They are all important!

Chest Discomfort

I am using the term *chest discomfort* intentionally rather than the term *chest pain* so that you will not think that your chest has to be painful in order for you to be experiencing an early symptom of a heart attack.

Chest discomfort may come during exercise or rest, day or night. It may begin in a mild form and, even over a period of one or two minutes, may increase, possibly spreading all the way across the chest, to be confused with muscle strain from overexertion. If there is no reason for muscle strain to have occurred, that is a clue that the discomfort may be a heart attack symptom. But even if there is a reason for muscle strain to occur, its abrupt onset still may be a symptom, and you should call your doctor to discuss it and see if you should proceed to the hospital. If your doctor is not available, go to the emergency room of your nearest hospital by the quickest available means.

Please note that chest discomfort may appear, then recede and even go away completely, and then may return. If you act within the first one or two minutes, you may experience this on your way to the hospital. *Just because chest discomfort may recede or vanish does not mean it is not a symptom and does not need attention.* Such transient episodes of discomfort, known as premonitory symptoms, are extremely important forewarnings and merit your getting treatment.

Again, remember that it is not necessary to experience persistent discomfort before you seek help. Many so-called sudden heart attacks are really not sudden but have begun with recognizable early warnings that can be heeded if you are aware of them.

Other Symptoms Sometimes Called the "Little-Known Signs of Heart Attacks"

Heart Discomfort in Parts of the Body Other than the Chest

Many people do not realize that heart attack discomfort very frequently extends into areas away from the front center of the chest or may occur in these other areas alone without being in the chest.

Understanding how discomfort happens in these other areas will help you to avoid making this serious mistake.

The reality is that pain messages from the chest may be read by the brain as coming from other areas. The reason has to do with the body's physiology. Messages of pain to the brain's pain center from the chest, arms, neck, jaws, and upper abdomen travel in separate nerve pathways until they approach the brain. Once there, the nerve channels converge and lie alongside each other. This close proximity permits pain signals to partly or completely cross over from the chest channel to one or more of the others. This causes the brain to misread the point of origin of discomfort so that its origin in the chest is incorrectly interpreted as coming from the arms, neck, jaws, or upper abdomen, or some combination thereof.

Arm Pain

In discussing arm pain, I use the term *pain* intentionally, because generally the early heart attack symptom that may occur in the arm is experienced as pain rather than discomfort (fig. 3.3). This does not mean that you should ignore arm discomfort as a possible sign, but the symptom may appear or progress to pain very rapidly.

Arm pain is usually experienced along the inner surface of the arm, the part nearest the body, but the pain may also involve the whole arm from the armpit downward or any individual part of it, such as the forearm or wrist. Arm pain is usually an ache but may be an unpleasant numbness or tingling. This pain, numbness, or tingling is most often in the left arm but may be in both arms or in only the right arm. It is crucial to know this, because many people believe it appears only in the left arm and therefore ignore right-arm pain or discomfort as an early warning sign.

Appearance of arm pain is frequently confused with arthritis, bursitis, or muscle strain. You can do a test yourself to see if these conditions are causing the pain. If moving your arm up and down aggravates the pain, it is not from your heart.

Nerve compression in the neck from arthritis of the spine or disc disease can cause pain extending down the arm that may also be confused with pain signaling a heart attack. You can usually recognize this as not being caused by the heart if turning your head or bending your neck aggravates it.

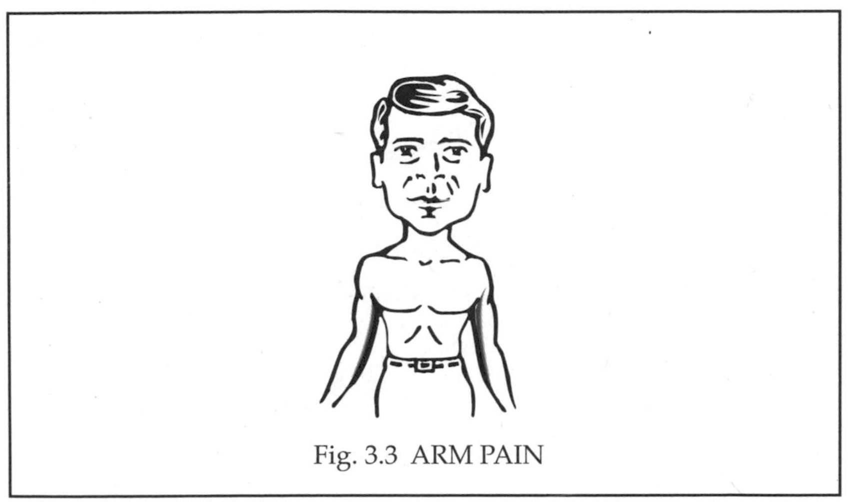

Fig. 3.3 ARM PAIN

Jaw and Neck Pain

Pain in the jaw or neck, or in both, is a very frequent symptom of heart attacks, and if it occurs, it may be more severe than chest discomfort (fig. 3.4). This can be confusing unless you realize the importance or jaw or neck pain or both as an early warning sign. This pain, which generally appears as an ache, may occur in conjunction with chest discomfort or separately, without any chest discomfort at all. It is impossible to estimate how many people have lost their lives through mistakenly seeking dental attention for their jaw ache instead of recognizing it as an early warning sign of a heart attack.

A Missouri patient, after reading one of the early-warning-sign articles based on our public education program, immediately called his doctor when jaw pain occurred. He reported that his "toothache" occurred even though he had false teeth. The doctor recognized that the toothache he described did not result from a dental condition and told him to go immediately to the emergency room, where he received prompt attention. The patient survived with very little heart damage.

One way to help you decide whether your pain is due to a bad tooth is to attempt to wiggle the painful tooth with your fingers, which will increase the pain caused by a bad tooth. Pain in the jaw signaling the onset of a heart attack is not worsened by wiggling a tooth. A number of dentists throughout Missouri have expressed

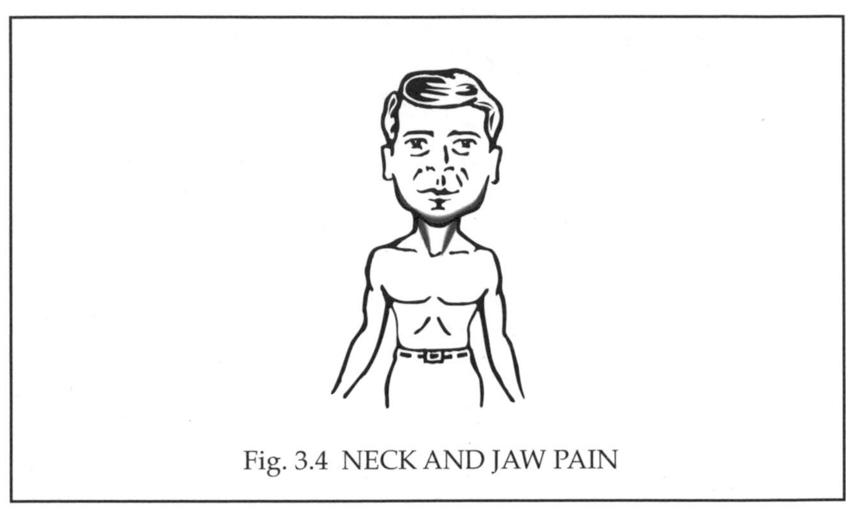

Fig. 3.4 NECK AND JAW PAIN

appreciation that their patients have been made aware of this serious type of jaw pain as a symptom of heart attacks through our public education campaign in the media.

Upper Abdominal Discomfort or Pain

A frequent topic in discussing heart attacks in women is the symptom of upper abdominal discomfort, which may be confused with indigestion (fig. 3.5). It is a frequent symptom in men as well. A six-month study of heart attack patient admissions to St. John's Hospital showed that 18 percent (nearly one in five) reported upper abdominal discomfort or pain as their chief symptom.[1]

This discomfort or pain is usually at the bottom of the rib cage at the forking of the ribs. It may be a downward extension of chest discomfort or may occur alone in the upper abdomen. It may be accompanied by nausea, and possibly by vomiting, making it easy for you to confuse it with such abdominal conditions as gallstones or hiatal hernia with gastroesophageal reflux disease (also known as acid reflux disease).

Making this all the more confusing is the fact that heart attacks frequently occur at night. When the symptoms occur after a large

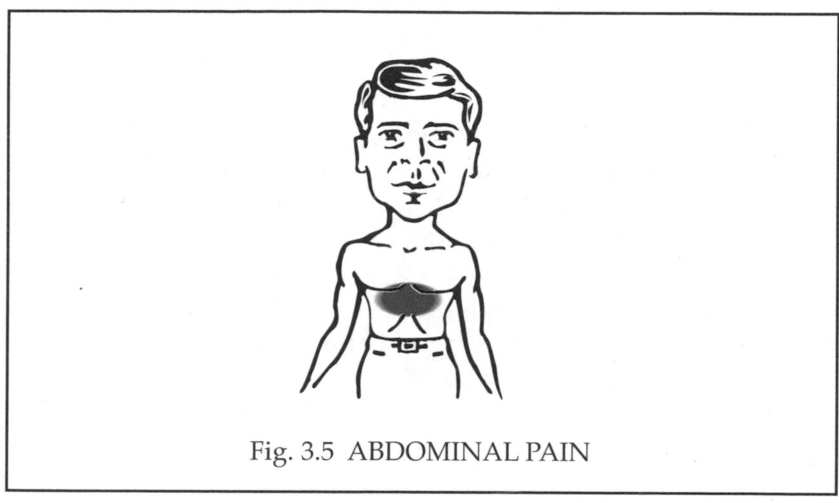
Fig. 3.5 ABDOMINAL PAIN

evening meal, blaming the distress on a hiatal hernia or just "plain indigestion" is especially easy. Doctors often tell of patients who had a heart attack in the middle of the night, who, not realizing it, tried unsuccessfully to relieve their distress with repeated doses of antacid and failed to survive until morning. What should you do about recognizing this symptom as an early warning sign of a heart attack?

First, if it is the first time you experience symptoms you believe are from "heartburn" (which is what acid reflux disease is often called), *do not* ignore it, and *do not* assume you know what it is. Call your doctor, even if it is in the middle of the night. It may signal that you need to get treated for a heart attack. If it turns out your doctor diagnoses it as acid reflux disease, you will get the medication and will begin to familiarize yourself with what it feels like when it occurs.

If you know you have acid reflux disease, it is still possible that you might experience upper abdominal discomfort or pain as an early warning sign of a heart attack. Unlike acid reflux disease, which is set off by "belching"—regurgitation of stomach contents—discomfort or pain in the upper abdomen from a heart attack is constant and not set off by belching. Nausea or vomiting may occur with either condition, so when in doubt, call your doctor.

Back Pain

Pain in the back is a common complaint, but it is not commonly known that back pain can be an early warning sign of a heart attack (fig. 3.6). Pain in the center of the chest may extend into the back or occur only in the back. It may occur anywhere above the waist, but usually it occurs between the shoulder blades. The six-month study of heart attack patients at St. John's Hospital showed that 13.6 percent reported back pain as a symptom.[2]

Back pain from a heart attack is usually an ache, often severe. Associated discomfort may occur elsewhere, especially pressure under the breastbone, but back pain may so overshadow discomfort in the front of the chest that you may fail to realize that the aching back may be caused by a heart attack, not by arthritis.

In the case of back pain, here is a tip that may be lifesaving: upon lying flat, heart attack pain in the back or elsewhere usually worsens, whereas arthritis or spine-fracture pain is usually diminished when lying down. Here is another test you can do: sit in a chair and bend forward, then straighten up again. Bending forward while seated and then straightening up almost always aggravates pain from arthritis or other trouble in the backbone, whereas heart attack pain is not affected by this action.

I am haunted by a story told to me by an eighty-year-old woman who came to St. John's suffering a heart attack, which she realized only after reading one of the articles generated by our early-warning-signs public education campaign. Describing her symptoms, she said that she had felt "an awful nagging pain between my shoulder blades every night for over a week when I went to bed, and it wasn't until I read today's paper that I realized I should come to the hospital." She died minutes later in my presence.

The disturbing frequency with which back pain from a heart attack goes unrecognized until it is too late illustrates the importance of learning and heeding this and the other early warning signs.

Discomfort in Combination

Two sites where discomfort frequently *but not always* appears in combination are the chest and possibly one or both arms and the chest and possibly the jaw or neck or both (fig. 3.7). I am repeating

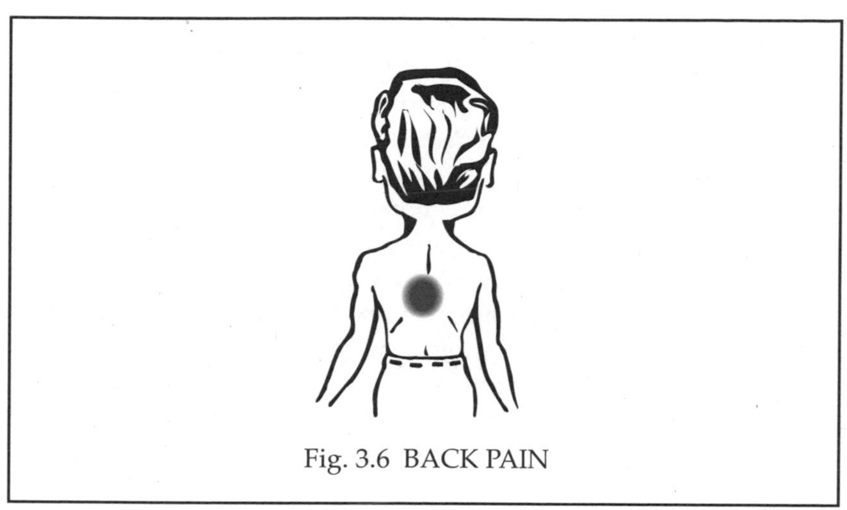

Fig. 3.6 BACK PAIN

these early warning signs that often appear in combination not only to emphasize their frequency but also to remind you that arm, jaw, or neck pain or a combination thereof may so overshadow chest discomfort—or appear without any chest discomfort—that the nature of an aching pain in the jaw or neck or one or both arms or a combination of these sites may be misinterpreted.

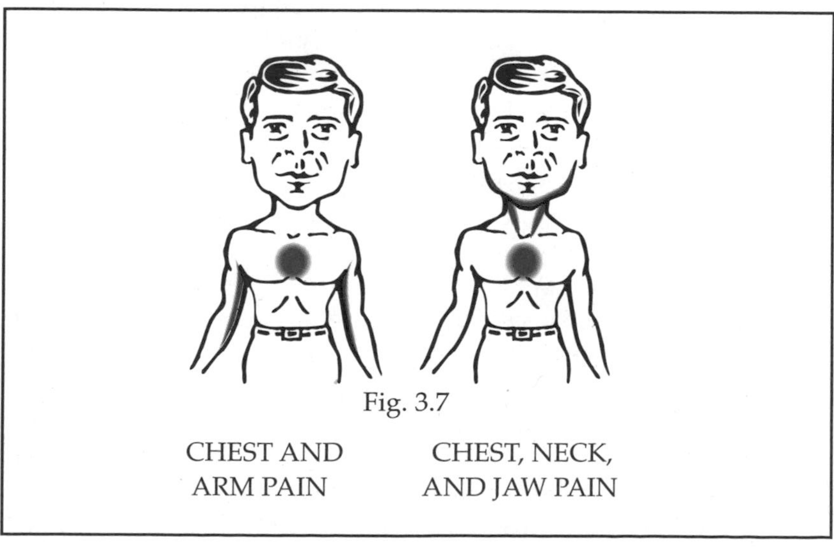

Fig. 3.7

CHEST AND ARM PAIN

CHEST, NECK, AND JAW PAIN

Other Equally Important Symptoms

Sweating

Sudden sweating, especially if heavy and without apparent cause, may be a symptom, and is experienced by 50 percent of patients with heart attacks (fig. 3.8). This sweating may soak your clothing, or it may be light. It is sometimes described as "breaking out in a cold sweat," but this is not necessarily correct, because the perspiration generally is not cold. *Unexplained sweating, with or without other symptoms, must always be evaluated.*

The newspaper reporter who wrote the first article about early warning signs in the *Springfield News Leader* told me about his own experience not recognizing sweating as a heart attack symptom. He said when his doctor took a routine ECG, the doctor discovered that he had had two previous heart attacks. The reporter could not recall pain or discomfort of any sort but clearly remembered having had two drenching sweats.

Shortness of Breath

Difficulty in breathing is a very frequent early warning sign and occurs by itself or in combination with other symptoms. You can usually tell that this shortness of breath is different from the shortness of breath from asthma, for example, which usually produces a wheezing in the chest. There is no wheezing from shortness of breath from heart attacks. Many have dangerously delayed seeking attention for a heart problem because they were unaware that shortness of breath is a frequent symptom of heart attacks.

Nausea

I mentioned nausea in association with upper abdominal discomfort or pain, but nausea may occur independently as a symptom, with or without vomiting. As with upper abdominal pain or discomfort, nausea is a symptom for which there are no easy answers since a number of common conditions cause it. This makes it all the more important that if you do not have a ready explanation, nausea should be considered a possible early warning sign of a heart attack.

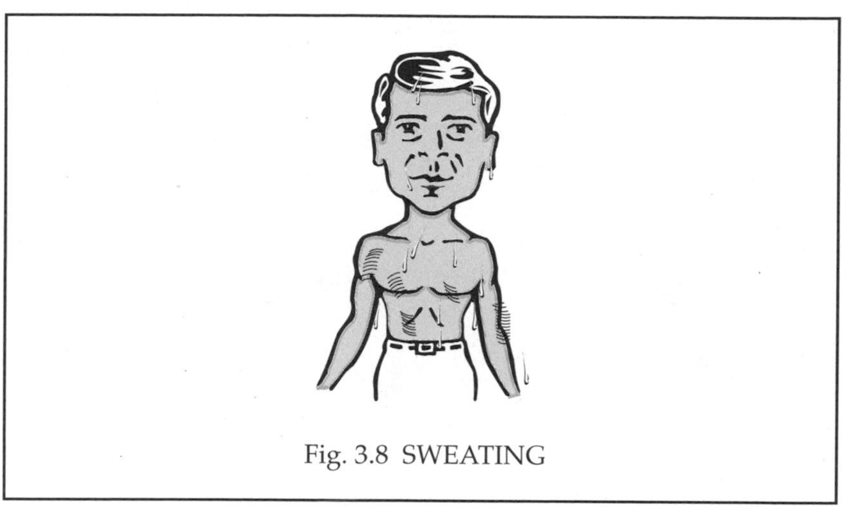

Fig. 3.8 SWEATING

An important rule of thumb is that even if you do have a hiatus hernia, acid reflux disease, or gallstones, if you wake up in the middle of the night with nausea, especially if upper abdominal pain is also present, you should consider the possibility that you are having a heart attack and immediately seek attention to find out. Sudden nausea can also occur as a heart attack symptom during the day.

Sudden Weakness

It is not generally known that suddenly becoming very weak may be an early warning sign of a heart attack. The cause for this is not well understood. Although weakness can come from many causes and is not always a reason for concern, sudden unexplained weakness needs careful attention and must immediately be checked out. Some doctors refer to this warning sign as "light-headedness."

"Painless" Heart Attacks

Doctors find an occasional patient with evidence of a previous heart attack for which no symptoms can be recalled. In these situations, it cannot be determined whether patients actually did not experience symptoms or whether symptoms were mild, the patient did

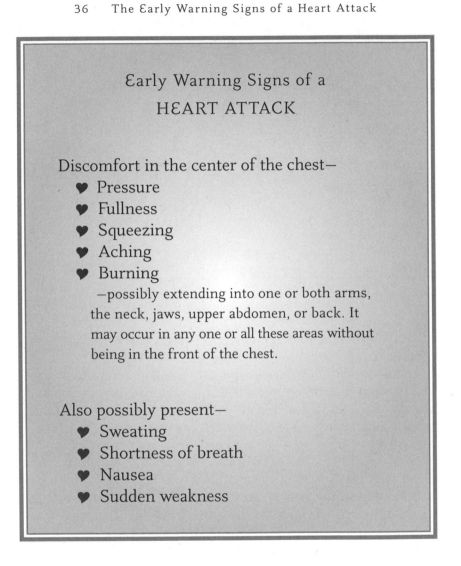

Early Warning Signs of a HEART ATTACK

Discomfort in the center of the chest—

- Pressure
- Fullness
- Squeezing
- Aching
- Burning

—possibly extending into one or both arms, the neck, jaws, upper abdomen, or back. It may occur in any one or all these areas without being in the front of the chest.

Also possibly present—

- Sweating
- Shortness of breath
- Nausea
- Sudden weakness

not recognize them as related to the heart, and he or she has subsequently forgotten them.

Since recognition and treatment of mild attacks are so crucial in avoiding later occurrence of more severe attacks, it is extremely important that you learn the full range of early warning signs and recognize that they vary in severity. It is also extremely important to have a yearly physical and request an ECG to make sure you have not had an unrecognized heart attack. *This advice is extremely important since the American Heart Association estimates that 175,000 "silent" heart attacks occur each year.*

Sudden Cardiac Arrest

Although I discussed sudden cardiac arrest due to ventricular fibrillation in the previous chapter as a complication of heart attacks and obviously it is not an early warning sign, I am bringing it up again here because, in many if not most cases, this catastrophic event results from failure to recognize and respond to the early warning signs. Cardiac arrest can happen very quickly. So I want to drive home to you the enormous value of learning and responding *immediately* to the appearance of any of the symptoms I have described by seeking immediate medical attention.

As I conducted the Missouri program, educating people about the early warning signs, some authorities told me that teaching these signs to people would not reduce the number of sudden cardiac deaths because such deaths occurred without forewarning. But my firsthand experience told me that this was an incorrect assumption. In conferences with the families of hundreds of patients who had expired suddenly, the majority told me that there had indeed been early heart warnings that had been mentioned but insufficiently recognized as important by both patient and family.

Inseparable from the topics of early warning signs and cardiac arrest is the great need for immediate response to a collapse from cardiac arrest. The first duty of anyone observing such a collapse is to immediately call 911 or the closest emergency response system. Next, you must start cardiopulmonary resuscitation (CPR) to sustain the patient until help arrives. Your most important action is once-per-second chest compression to sustain circulation until electrical defibrillation can be carried out. The traditional mouth-to-mouth breathing has recently been abandoned because it is of no benefit, actually interfering with the vital maintenance of circulation by the closed-chest heart massage. This service, essential for survival, especially preservation of brain function, must be provided by bystanders close at hand since ambulance paramedics rarely can get there in less than several minutes.

To shorten the interval to availability of a defibrillator, public-access automatic external defibrillators (AEDs) are increasingly being placed in locations where people congregate, such as shopping malls, sites of athletic events, office buildings, and airplanes. Their use requires that individuals in those locations be trained to use them properly. Without this combination of bystander CPR and prompt defibrillation, survival after out-of-hospital cardiac arrest is extremely low. Splendid training in CPR and AED use is provided by the American Heart Association, the American Red Cross, and other heart-related service groups. Another major advance is the widespread use of implanted automatic defibrillators in those found to be at high risk of cardiac arrest. Many thousands of these are installed each year in the United States.

This chapter about how to recognize and respond promptly to the early warning signs of a heart attack and later chapters about treatment choices and lifetime preventive measures make this a handbook of how to avoid many preventable heart attacks and how to reduce deaths and disability from those that do occur.

Remember what we have taught in our Missouri public education program: *Sudden death from a heart attack is often really not sudden. Know the warning signs!*

CHAPTER 4

Heart Attack or Angina?

Angina is an illness experienced by many thousands that has symptoms identical to those of a heart attack except for the circumstances of occurrence, severity, and duration (fig. 4.1). It is caused by narrowing of the coronary arteries preventing adequate blood flow downstream during times of increased need. This need commonly results from physical exertion but may also be from emotional stress, an excessively rapid heartbeat, or blood loss. If the need comes from exertion, it usually subsides within five minutes of ceasing the exertion, more rapidly if nitroglycerin is placed under the tongue. If the need arises during emotional stress or excitement, it may persist until relaxation occurs. If angina results from an excessively rapid heartbeat, treatment to interrupt the rapid beating is needed because continuation can result in heart damage downstream.

By contrast, heart attack discomfort may occur during exercise or rest, day or night. If it occurs during exercise, it does not cease upon stopping exertion. It is usually prolonged and is more likely to be associated with sweating.

If you have not developed angina, it is vital for you to understand it so that if you experience symptoms, you can recognize them early and get treatment. If you have angina, you need to know that its abrupt worsening often indicates the beginning of a heart attack. You can tell that it is worsening if discomfort occurs with less exertion or even when you are at rest, or if discomfort is more severe than it has been, lasts longer, or responds more slowly to nitroglycerin. This

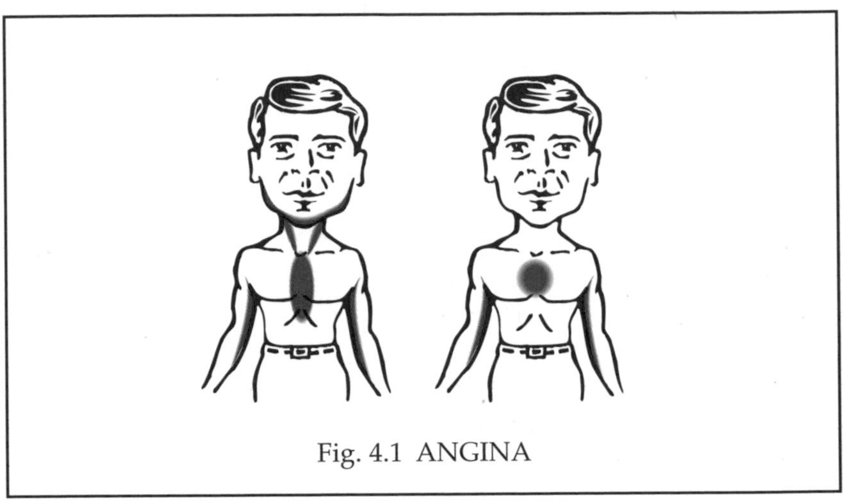

Fig. 4.1 ANGINA

change is usually due to a disruption of a deposit of cholesterol and the beginning of blood clot formation.

The result was once called unstable angina but is now usually referred to as acute coronary syndrome, or ACS, the term I discussed in Chapter 2 that is also used in other heart disease contexts. If an intensifying of angina occurs, call your doctor immediately. If your doctor is not available promptly, get to a hospital emergency room. Many people have sustained heart attacks, some fatal, as a result of not knowing they should respond to this change. The frequency with which acute coronary syndrome progresses to a heart attack is now widely known by physicians, and these episodes are getting a vast amount of attention in emergency rooms.

Another point that is important for you to understand is that whereas angina is a chronic condition, all cases have an acute beginning. By this I mean that there is a point at which a person developing angina experiences the discomfort I have described for the first time. Although most angina probably occurs as a result of the gradual narrowing of coronary arteries by cholesterol deposits, I am convinced that some angina starts as the result of the beginning of blood clots that have not advanced sufficiently to cause heart attacks. Thus, if you learn the symptoms of angina and how to recognize them at the earliest stage, should they occur you can save your life and prevent disability.

CHAPTER 5

How to Get Proper—and Prompt—Treatment for a Heart Attack

You have learned how your heart functions, what a heart attack is, and how to identify the early warning signs that will tell you that you need to seek care. In this chapter you will learn how to obtain the care you need and how to obtain it as quickly as possible. Much of the information currently being disseminated to potential heart attack patients—and that is everyone—about how to proceed if heart attack warning signs appear is incorrect and is costing lives. One of my major purposes in writing this book is to rectify this deplorable situation. The first issue I want to look at is how someone experiencing one or more of the early warning signs can best get care as quickly as possible.

As I mentioned, on its inception the Missouri program yielded the startling result of cutting almost in half the four hours that previously were required by patients and their families to decide to start to the hospital after the onset of heart attack symptoms. It also increased by 60 percent the admissions of patients with actual or threatened heart attacks to the cardiovascular care unit. The key points from our program that are vital to your own prompt recognition and response to symptoms are:

* *Know* the full range of symptoms at their earliest point, even when they are subtle or intermittent—*and if you believe you are experiencing a symptom, immediately chew a full-size uncoated aspirin.*

- *Follow* this advice: If you experience any of these warning signs, call your doctor, and if he or she is not immediately available, get to the hospital emergency room.
- *Get* to the hospital by the fastest means possible. We did not specify mode of transport but left this decision to the judgment of the physician and patient. We recognized that many patients dislike traveling by ambulance and prefer the family automobile, which we knew to be quicker and remarkably safe. (In fact, as I will discuss later in this chapter, research has shown that patients' choice to use car transportation is in almost all cases prudent.)

These three points are crucial to getting prompt care for a heart attack. The last two points are the reasons I so strongly disagree with the prevailing national policy, started by the American Heart Association in the mid-1970s, of calling 911 if heart attack symptoms occur. This policy has become so ingrained in our culture that you might not even recognize it as a policy; it just seems to be a given, and for that reason it may have acquired an air of authority. I am going to analyze and critique this policy to remove all doubt about what you should do in a heart attack emergency.

I mentioned in the Introduction that there has never been a nationwide public education campaign about the early warning signs of heart attacks. Except for Southwest Missouri, where, under the auspices of the Hammons Heart Institute and then the Turner Heart Foundation, we conducted an intensive early-warning-signs public and professional educational program, the national void in providing this lifesaving information lasted until the mid-1990s. During that time, American cardiologists were predominantly occupied with developing and using the remarkable new advances in treating heart attack patients *after* they arrived at the hospital.

In 1994, the National Heart, Lung, and Blood Institute (NHLBI), acting on its desire to create a national educational program to get heart attack patients to the hospital sooner, launched the Rapid Early Action for Coronary Treatment (REACT) program as a test study. You have probably never heard of REACT, but it is common for studies known only to the medical community to have a ripple effect on the public at large from the conclusions that find their way into the media. Thus, it is worth looking at REACT, because even if you have not heard of it, REACT may actually have affected your assumptions about heart care. This point is important because, as you will see, what the program attempted to communicate about getting treatment for heart attacks was deeply flawed.

The dual objective of this sixteen million–dollar program, sponsored by the largest U.S. federal agency dedicated to heart issues, was to test the "effect of a community intervention on patient delay and emergency medical services use in acute coronary heart diseases."[1] In other words, REACT's designers wanted to see if they could cut down patient delay in arriving at emergency rooms and increase use of ambulances.

Exhaustive studies explored how patients made medical decisions and why these decisions were frequently delayed in cases of a heart attack. Reports of eight studies were assembled to justify the REACT conclusion that calling one's doctor in case of a heart attack delays care. This is a critical point and flies in the face of what I have advised you to do. But does calling your doctor actually delay care?

Reviewing the studies cited by REACT shows that five of them were from other countries where medical care systems are not comparable to those in the United States.[2] Thus, the studies that concluded that calling a doctor delays patient care are inapplicable in the United States. The three reports from the United States were from older studies,[3] and are not convincing to me because they lacked the accuracy of the Missouri data, which found that patients' calling their personal physicians facilitated their getting prompt care.

Further impacting the question about whether to call your doctor if heart attack symptoms occur are comments made by personal physicians to REACT's designers prior to the program's launch. As part of REACT's data gathering on heart care, numerous personal physicians were interviewed (61 percent of them were internists; 35 percent were family practitioners). These doctors expressed great pride in their knowledge of their patients, and they thought that if heart attack symptoms appeared, their patients' first call should be to them because they could give advice tailored to the patient.[4] Rather than incorporating this point of view into the plan for their program, REACT's designers chose to ignore the doctors' suggestion.

As part of the REACT program, four months were spent gathering patient data on heart attack symptom onset to hospital arrival time and ambulance use in ten pairs of matched (similar) communities in five states. This was followed by an intensive eighteen-month public education news-media campaign in one community of each pair to see if REACT's messages could get possible heart attack sufferers in communities where the campaign was conducted to the hospital more quickly than those in the other communities.[5] According to its own report at the program's conclusion, the way the public education campaign was conducted was flawed, and in comparison with the ten communities where the campaign was not conducted, REACT failed to hasten hospital arrival time for those experiencing a heart attack.

REACT's flawed messages are worth looking at because they did not get people to the hospital more quickly in heart emergencies, so they present an example of what *does not* work. I want you to be clear about this so that in a possible heart emergency you will not be confused about what does not work and concentrate on what does. That way you will get to the hospital sooner.

These were REACT's flaws:

- Ignoring people's dislike of travel by ambulance, REACT sought to hasten patient hospital arrival and to increase hospital admissions by increasing 911 ambulance use through promoting calling 911 for heart emergencies.
- REACT paid virtually no attention to *early* heart attack warnings. Patients were advised to call for help if symptoms persisted for more than fifteen minutes after onset, meaning that they should not call sooner. The "onset" of symptoms was defined as the point at which mild symptoms became more severe. The time from the actual onset of symptoms to the point of worsening is often appreciable. Adding this time to the fifteen minutes REACT told patients to wait creates a further delay and amounts to a total period of time during which many deaths occur. This program policy was terribly wrong. As I explained in Chapter 3 when I detailed the early warning signs, an adequately informed person can usually tell within one or two minutes after the actual beginning of even mild symptoms that something is wrong.
- In keeping with its instruction to wait at least fifteen minutes and to wait for symptoms to worsen, REACT's news-media portrayals of discomfort patterns were inadequate and more in keeping with *late* rather than *early* heart attack signs.

* REACT gave very little attention to the extremely important symptoms I have described as the little-known signs of heart attacks, which consist of discomfort in areas other than the chest. All of REACT's data were gathered on the basis of "chest pain."
* REACT's strong public dictum that all patients with a possible heart attack travel to the hospital only by 911 ambulance implies the seriously mistaken, if unspoken, advice to bypass the extremely important personal physician and the family automobile, which is often the quickest, as well as the most comfortable, mode of transportation to the hospital;

These were REACT's failed results:

* The delay of coronary heart disease patients in reaching the hospital was not reduced.
* The number of coronary heart disease patients admitted to the hospital did not increase.
* The program produced no reduction in coronary heart disease deaths.
* The use of 911 ambulance services by coronary heart disease patients remained almost unchanged despite the eighteen-month intensive news-media campaign advocating an increase. In my opinion, this reflects that across the United States, patients with possible heart attacks are reluctant or unwilling to travel by ambulance, the majority preferring to use the family automobile.

I had hoped that REACT's failure would have caused the NHLBI and the AHA to abandon "911 for all heart attacks," but both are continuing to promote this policy—which is why I am discussing it here. As a doctor, I am far from alone in urging a rethinking of this policy. In fact, REACT reported that in its interviews with personal physicians prior to the program's launch, "a substantial proportion" of the doctors "questioned the appropriateness of 911 use." There were also comments that patients preferred to travel by car and disliked going by ambulance. Clearly, these statements were ignored by REACT and are still being ignored by the NHLBI and the AHA in their advocacy of "911 for all."

This brings us to the core question: What should *you* do if you are experiencing the early warning signs of a heart attack? Should you call your doctor, go to the hospital on your own, or call 911?

You may remember that in Chapter 3 I told you to call your doctor or, if your doctor is not available, go to the hospital by the quickest means possible. Because messages that contradict this advice appear in the media, you may still be confused, or at least ambivalent, about which course to take. Since speed is of the utmost importance, you need to fix clearly in your mind *exactly* what your most effective course of action would be in this life-threatening circumstance.

Research shows that the greatest portion of the excessively long period from the onset of heart attack symptoms to hospital arrival is taken up by delay of the patient and family deciding to seek help.[6] Only a small part of this period is occupied by getting to the hospital after you decide to go, but your decision-making process and your decisions during this time are extremely important.

It is my belief that if you developed possible heart attack symptoms, the majority of you, even without reading this book, would first call your doctor or go on your own to the hospital by car. My purpose here is to reinforce the correctness of this judgment so that you will make this decision *immediately*. I want to eliminate the background "buzz" of contradictory information that might waste time by slowing down your decision-making process. With the wide dissemination of the "911 for all" directive, I am certain that in the midst of a heart emergency many people waste perhaps considerable time deciding whether to reject that advice. I want to eliminate this delay.

As you know, I have recommended that, if possible, on first experiencing an early warning sign of a heart attack, you call your doctor. I have reported to you the effective participation of personal physicians in the Missouri program to hasten patient arrival. I have also mentioned the strong and convincing, albeit ignored, interest in heart attack care expressed by personal physicians interviewed in the five states of the REACT study. During my decades of practice as a cardiologist I have had extremely fruitful associations with scores of family practitioners and general internist personal physicians and was highly impressed with their day-and-night attention to their patients.

Deciding to involve your personal physician in a heart emergency requires the following:

- You must have a health insurance policy that allows you to call your doctor in case of an emergency.

- You must have a doctor to whom you can comfortably relate and who will see you for checkups at suitable intervals throughout the year so that he or she gains a thorough knowledge of your overall health and medical conditions.
- You must find out whether your doctor wants to participate in a heart emergency or would prefer that instead you call 911. If it is the latter, I suggest you change doctors (see Chapter 6).
- If your doctor does want to be involved in a possible heart emergency, ascertain how you can make immediate day or night contact with him or her (or a doctor on standby). Explain that you realize that in heart emergencies you cannot wait for a return call and would get to a hospital.

If you experience the early warning signs of a heart attack, what advantages does calling your personal physician give you (fig. 5.1)? A call to your doctor can quickly remove any uncertainty about whether you should go to the hospital, saving you time. Your doctor can recognize noncardiac symptoms, sparing you an unnecessary emergency trip to the hospital. If you do need to go, your doctor can tell you which hospital you should go to and discuss with you the best means of getting there. Your doctor may tell you to have a friend or family member drive you or, if no one is available, to drive yourself. If symptoms are more severe, your doctor may tell you to call 911. In my practice, when patients calling me needed an ambulance, I made the call to 911, giving instructions to the paramedics and directing them to cut short or eliminate the usually wasteful "stabilization at the scene" time. (I will explain later why I usually consider this to be wasted time.)

Regardless of your mode of transportation, your doctor can notify the ER of your impending arrival, giving the staff vital information about your health, which, in my experience, most doctors remember remarkably well. Your doctor can then join you at the hospital, with important early involvement in your care. At the ER, you will be taken care of by an emergency physician, and, in many cases, a cardiologist will be on call.

Of the patients who call their doctors prior to arriving at the ER, I am not aware of any research that shows how many are directed to travel by car versus ambulance. In the research done as part of the Missouri program, the fact that the great majority of patients called

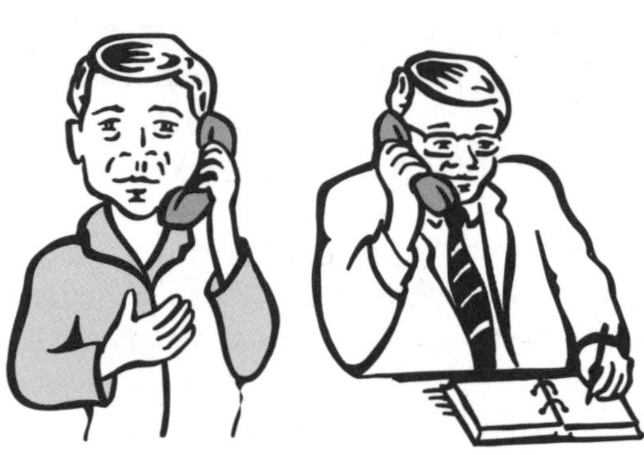

Fig. 5.1

If you experience any of the early warning signs, **call your doctor** day or night. If he or she is not available, get to the hospital emergency room. Upon receiving your call, your personal physician can take charge and expedite attention to your emergency.

their doctors as their first step in seeking help during a period when ambulance use was decreasing suggests that the physicians favored travel by car.

This brings us to the second vital question: Should you go by car, either on direction from your doctor or, if your doctor is not available, on your own initiative? I strongly recommend that you go to the ER by car unless there is an actual need for an ambulance. The car is quicker than using 911 and, as mentioned, is generally remarkably safe. A major study in Salt Lake City showed that heart attack patients traveling by private means reached the hospital twenty-nine minutes sooner than those going by paramedic-staffed mobile coronary care units.[7] Another study showed that serious difficulty before hospital arrival occurred in 0.3 percent of patients coming by car versus 5.6 percent of those using an ambulance, an incidence almost nineteen times greater.[8] Of the 0.3 percent of patients coming by car who experienced serious difficulty, half experienced these difficulties before being placed by family members in the car, and, therefore, would have experienced these difficulties if they had chosen to go by ambulance, which would have arrived even later. This study showed that the great majority of patients who traveled by car made the choice prudently.

I am convinced that there is far less psychological stress in calling your doctor or in deciding on your own to go to the hospital than there is in making an unpleasant 911 decision—and this means deciding more quickly. Traveling in the family automobile is also much less emotionally stressful than going by ambulance. I have had a number of patients whose conditions worsened severely in ambulances because of the ambulances' use of sirens and rapid speed.

If your doctor does wish to be involved in your acute care, discuss the choice of transportation in the event of an emergency. Since you know from reading this book that the majority of heart attack patients travel by car unless severely ill, it is very appropriate for you to express that preference also. Many of my patients were quick to voluntarily tell me that they did not want to go to the hospital by ambulance. But when you call your doctor about possible early warning signs—or in a prior discussion with your doctor about what to do in case of a heart attack emergency—if your doctor recommends ambulance transportation, *follow your doctor's instructions.*

We are now at the third vital question: Under what circumstances, other than by instruction of your doctor, should you call 911? This valuable service should be reserved for people truly in need—mostly those who feel or appear to be severely ill. This includes people who have collapsed or appear likely to collapse on the basis of faintness, reduction in consciousness, or shortness of breath, since paramedics can carry out resuscitation measures at the site.

It is important to note that if you are obviously very ill and can arrive at the hospital by car sooner than an ambulance could reach your home, you should take the car. Scores of my dangerously ill patients have been brought to the hospital by car. I cannot recall a single mishap on the way, nor can I recall any difficulty on the way to the hospital for the hundreds of less ill patients I treated who traveled by car.

There are other circumstances where 911 service is needed. The most frequent is in the case of people who live alone and have no one nearby to drive them. Notwithstanding widespread advice to the contrary, countless patients who live alone and have no one else to drive them do drive themselves.[9] If you live alone, I suggest talking to a family member or friend about being available to drive you in case of an emergency. Talk to two people so that you will have a backup if one is unavailable.

Since the decision about transportation is so crucial, I want to give you a clear picture of the value and the limitations of the vital 911 emergency transport system (EMS) in acute heart attack care. This system originated in the early 1970s with the introduction of the "mobile coronary care unit," which was essentially an intensive care unit on wheels. The original concept was to bring this unit to the patient at the site of illness and to "stabilize the patient at the scene," permitting unhurried transportation to the hospital after this stabilization was accomplished.

Soon, some experts expressed the opinion that spending this time before starting to the hospital did not improve patient care, but the practice continued. Missouri governor Warren Hearnes appointed me as the cardiologist member of his Technical Advisory Committee on Emergency Medical Communication, the first step in establishing Missouri's 911 system. I also served as a consultant to the state legislature in drafting training and certification standards for paramedics and emergency medical technicians, and participated in their training in Southwest Missouri. Later I went to Seattle, a pioneer city in ambulance transportation, to study their EMS system, riding in an ambulance on calls.

I mention this so that you will know I spent more than three decades of work in developing a 911 EMS system in the Southwest Missouri region, and that I believe it is a lifesaving service *when appropriately used.* Nevertheless, as I have stated, I have significant concerns about the advocacy of 911 EMS service for all heart attacks rather than for people who are severely ill. I want to spell out my concerns to make it crystal clear to you *why* calling 911 creates unnecessary delays for non–severely ill patients. First, a 911 call leads to two-way ambulance travel (from the base station to the patient's home and from there to the hospital), which takes more time than the one-way travel by car from the home to the hospital. Second, you must add the time required to reach the patient's home to the time required to mobilize the ambulance attendants. At night, when the staff may not be awake and dressed, and, in some regions, may be sleeping away from their station, this time may be considerable. Third, a frequent delay, especially in rural but sometimes in metropolitan areas, caused by difficulty of the driver in locating a residence, is extremely frightening to a patient who is waiting for the ambulance (and to the doctor who is waiting at the ER for patient arrival). At times I have had the family post one member along the way to guide the ambulance into the driveway, or, in the city, to identify for the driver the patient's house or apartment. Fourth, the persistence of the apparently ingrained, and to me very disturbing, EMS policy of carrying out the "stabilization of the patient at the scene" adds additional time. One report, from Maryland, reported twenty-two minutes as the average time at the scene.[10] St. John's Hospital in Springfield reported that time at the scene averaged twenty minutes.[11] This time is spent taking a history, doing a physical examination, and installing an intravenous line. Unless active resuscitation (that is, CPR) or other urgently needed treatment is needed, such as for breathing difficulty, I believe that these functions should be carried out at the hospital. An extremely brief examination, taking no more than a minute or two, will usually suffice. The widely disseminated claim that a 911 call brings heart care to you quickly at your home is a serious overstatement. Either by car or by ambulance, you can usually be in your local hospital emergency room and under the care of a physician and staff more expert than the highly trained paramedic and emergency medical technician in less time than is usually spent at your home. I have already noted that if you go by car to the emergency room, an ECG can be performed in less than eight minutes; if you go by ambulance, an ECG can be recorded and transmitted while you are in transit. Recent concerns have been raised about the problems involved in prehospital administration of thrombolysis by paramedics. Indeed, Dr. W. Douglas Weaver, division head of cardiovascular medicine at the Henry Ford Hospital in Detroit, observed that EMS services in the United States are "fragmented" (meaning that they are not universally organized and functional).[12] And last, my patients' dislike of riding in an ambulance sends a clear message to me: if people believe they should call 911 in case of a possible heart attack, many will delay making this unpleasant call until it is absolutely necessary, not realizing that by this time the illness will be more severe or they may even die.

To summarize the points I have covered thus far: If you have a heart attack, your survival and reduction of disability depend on learning the early warning signs, responding promptly, and knowing how to respond promptly. This allows you to get to the hospital in time to take advantage of treatments that are lifesaving if given soon enough. I have explained how to accomplish this and why, if possible, involving your doctor in this process is important.

To save your life and prevent or minimize disability, keep this in mind: *By far, your best chance of getting treatment under way within the first sixty minutes of symptoms (the golden hour) is to go immediately by car if your doctor advises it—or, if your doctor is unavailable, on your own initiative—to your nearest hospital, or, if you are severely ill, to immediately call 911.* This action also greatly improves your chance of getting the substantial benefits of treatment administered before the end of the third hour of symptoms, at which time benefits drop sharply.

How to Get Prompt Treatment When You Get to the Emergency Room

As part of the heavy emphasis in promoting 911 use, you may have heard that in order to get prompt treatment at the ER, you should go there by ambulance rather than by car. In fact, this was a formal recommendation of REACT in a report in the *American Heart Journal* in January 2004.[13] My response to this belief is that it is wrong. The very small study used as the basis for saying that patients who travel by ambulance get more prompt treatment was seriously flawed. There was no attempt made at the hospital to record how many of these patients were seriously ill, which would have necessarily hastened treatment whether patients arrived by ambulance or car. There was also no report of how many patients expired, a very reliable measure of illness severity.

I noted earlier a report showing that more severely ill patients tend to take ambulances, as indicated by the high frequency of cardiac arrest during ambulance transportation compared with arrests during automobile transportation.[14] Even more compelling was another report that of all the heart attack patients admitted to the 1,674 hospitals in the National Registry of Myocardial Infarction, the death rate in the hospital in those arriving by ambulance was 14.3 percent versus 5.5 percent in patients arriving by car, indicating the ambulance patients to be "very sick."[15]

My analysis is that severely ill patients very appropriately travel by ambulance and that regardless of whether severely ill patients come by ambulance or car, ER staffs have the duty of attending more severely ill patients ahead of those who are less ill.

What should you expect, and how should you conduct yourself, if, in a heart emergency, you arrive at an emergency room by car? I am going to describe a situation in which your personal physician is not available to meet you. Calling your personal physician and having him or her there will facilitate the process.

Although ERs, often now referred to as emergency departments (EDs), have come to be heavily burdened by nonemergencies, vigorous national campaigning by the NHLBI has markedly improved the reception and management of potential heart emergencies. After getting out of your car and leaving it with the door attendant, you will first come to the reception (or triage) desk, usually staffed by a nurse. You should tell the nurse in an assertive tone, "I think I am having a heart attack and must be seen immediately." If necessary, pound on the desk! This will probably cut short any detailed interrogation about your symptoms.

It is not correct procedure for the receptionist to refute your statement. If you are not taken inside at once, you need to say that you must see a doctor right away. This will usually be effective. *Do not hesitate to speak forcefully—it is your life at stake!* The days of unnecessary deaths from heart attacks in the ER, portrayed in the 1971 film *The Hospital,* are over. Refuse to complete registration and insurance papers, leaving that to whoever brought you; if you have come alone, defer it until your care is under way.

Inside, you must be seen by a doctor and a nurse, who may need to be interrupted at another task, since your problem is likely to be more important than almost any other except arterial bleeding. As the doctor is examining you, an ECG machine and operator should arrive at your side. An ECG tracing should be made and interpreted within ten minutes of your arrival (fig. 5.2). Research shows that the nationwide average for accomplishing this is nine minutes.[16] The fact that this is being accomplished now in most hospitals is evidence that the national efforts to expedite care are paying off.

If a heart attack has occurred, the doctor, after rapidly learning your medical history, doing a physical examination, and performing the ECG, will usually yield the diagnosis within fifteen minutes of your arrival. Meanwhile, your pain or discomfort will have been relieved by intravenous morphine. In this usually highly organized

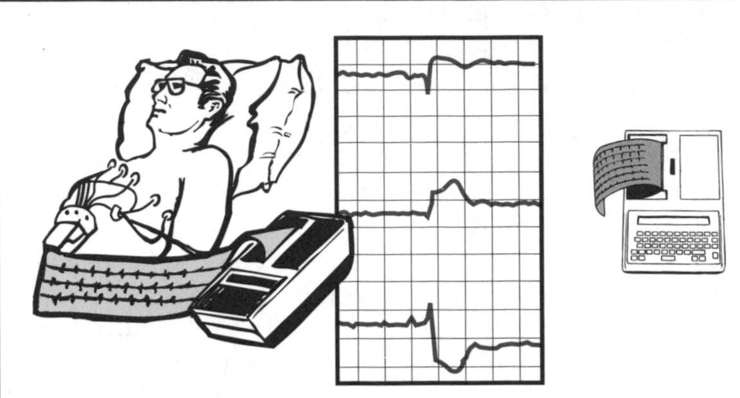

Fig. 5.2 ECG

An immediate ECG, or heart tracing, ideally within **ten minutes** of hospital arrival, is crucial to early institution of lifesaving care. ECG of a major heart attack in a forty-six-year-old woman, stopped in the first sixty minutes by thrombolysis in her community hospital eighty-five miles from Springfield. She did not sustain any heart damage.

fashion, definitive treatment can be started in fifteen to thirty minutes of your reaching the ER.

If you, a family member, or a friend does not receive the promptness of attention I have described, if it is during the day *immediately alert the hospital administrator.* This will surely bring about a change in the staff's responsiveness to your needs. If it is after office hours, continue being insistent. After you get treatment and are safely home, write a "letter to the editor" of your newspaper. I can assure you that hospitals pay attention to such letters, because if they do not correct inefficient practices, they will lose business!

What Treatments Are Available to You?

If a heart attack is diagnosed, a prompt choice of treatment needs to be made. Unless instant treatment is mandatory, the doctor should briefly explain to you the available options so that you can accept or reject the recommended plan. This process of getting your approval is known as gaining "informed consent," and is universally required before surgical operations.

Since your need for treatment might come unexpectedly, I am going to provide you with information so that you will be better able to participate in an informed-consent discussion. Here, I will present an overview of the treatments; in subsequent chapters, I will discuss them in more detail to help you make choices.

Thrombolysis

This is the breakthrough treatment I referred to in the Introduction that can "stop a heart attack in its tracks." In this treatment, "clot buster" medications that dissolve the blood clots that cause heart attacks are injected into a vein. Throughout the country, this treatment can be begun within fifteen to thirty minutes of your arrival at the ER. If given during the first sixty minutes of symptoms, the death rate is cut in half.

As blood clots age, they become more difficult to dissolve, but if thrombolysis can be given before the end of the third hour of symptoms, deaths can be reduced by 25 percent. After three hours, by which time the death of heart muscle resulting from the attack is usually complete, this and other treatments are less effective.

Patients who have recently had surgery, who have a body injury that might cause bleeding, or who have had a recent stroke and those with very high blood pressure, unless that can be promptly corrected in the emergency room, are not eligible for thrombolysis.

Balloon Coronary Artery Angioplasty

The first step in determining whether balloon coronary artery angioplasty is needed is angiography (see Chapter 8), which takes photographs of the coronary arteries, disclosing blockages. If angiography indicates that balloon angioplasty is needed, the next step is coronary angioplasty.

Coronary angioplasty consists of inserting a slender tube, a catheter, with a collapsed balloon at the tip into an artery at the groin or in the arm, then passing it upward and inserting it into the opening of the obstructed coronary artery. The catheter's balloon tip is then introduced into the artery and inserted into the clot. The balloon is then inflated, compressing the soft clot and reopening the artery.

The diagnostic coronary angiography can be done only in major hospitals (technically known as tertiary hospitals) that have a cardiac catheterization laboratory, or cath lab. Of the 4,942 acute-care hospitals in the United States, only 1,588 have a cath lab. All of these labs are equipped for diagnosis, but only 1,202 are *interventional* cath labs, equipped and staffed to provide balloon angioplasty,[17] and some of these do not offer it at night.

Although the NHLBI has recommended getting the balloon inserted within 90 minutes of the patient's arrival at the ER,[18] it has recently been reported that only 30 percent of hospitals achieve this goal.[19] The average delay at one major hospital promoting angioplasty is 120 minutes, or 2 hours.[20] Adding this to the average 2.7-hour delay in hospital arrival already discussed means that patients getting balloon treatment may receive it at nearly five hours after the onset of symptoms, well beyond the three-hour point at which treatment becomes much less effective.

To bridge the interval between ER arrival and insertion of the balloon, there have been extensive trials of administering thrombolysis on arrival, with balloon angioplasty as soon as possible thereafter. But this has not become standard practice, because the combination causes excessive bleeding during the cath lab procedure.

Various trials combining thrombolysis on arrival followed by later balloon angioplasty in cases where symptoms persist are still under way. I will perform an in-depth analysis of thrombolysis in Chapter 7 and of balloon angioplasty in Chapter 9.

Regardless of the treatment plan, a number of drugs are standard:

- an adult-size uncoated aspirin on arrival, to be chewed (unless, as I have advised, you have taken one before leaving for the ER)
- heparin, or a variant, the drug derived from leeches, which interrupts the clotting of blood but does not dissolve clots
- beta-blockers, to reduce the work of the heart
- antiplatelet agents, especially clopidogril (Plavix) and the IIB/IIIA inhibitors

* medication to reduce or increase blood pressure and to regulate heart rhythm as needed
* morphine intravenously, which is standard for pain relief

For patients not eligible for thrombolysis and those for whom balloon angioplasty is not elected, the foregoing medications are of great value.

This overview of treatment choices shows why you need to recognize heart attack symptoms early and quickly and get to your *nearest* hospital for treatment, during the first hour of symptoms—the golden hour—or within the next two hours. Make sure you get thrombolysis, if you are eligible. Reserve your right to choose another treatment later, regardless of whether that later treatment will be at the local hospital you have come to because it is nearer or, if balloon angioplasty is indicated, a tertiary hospital with a cath lab and interventional cardiologists to do the procedure.

Although I will focus in detail on thrombolysis and balloon angioplasty in Chapters 7 and 9, in this overview I want to be emphatic about your priorities: Your goal is getting to the *nearest* hospital, not to the biggest hospital. Most patients are eligible for thrombolysis, and local hospitals can administer it quickly. Later, when balloon angioplasty is considered, you can elect to transfer to a tertiary hospital. Angiography may reveal that you do not need balloon angioplasty. Many patients who have received thrombolysis do not need balloon angioplasty. Although balloon angioplasty can generally be done safely three days after thrombolysis, current research indicates that it is not effective when performed three days or later after a heart attack (see Chapter 9). In my view, this is a major finding, because until recently angioplasty has been overprescribed. Even patients who were successfully treated with thrombolysis were often given angioplasty because it was assumed to be effective.

You can see how vital it is for you to be clear about exercising your prerogatives in the emergency room. Remember my comments about informed consent: In acute heart care, except in instant emergencies, you are always entitled to informed consent. You and you alone have the right to make these lifesaving decisions. The major goal of this book is to provide you with the information you need to make the decisions.

CHAPTER 6

How to Choose and Work with a Personal Physician (and the Patient's Bill of Rights)

In today's environment of managed care and health insurance that restrict some patients' options, it is not always possible to have personal doctors available in emergencies. Many plans do allow it, however, and for this reason I want to examine in some detail the role of the personal doctor in heart care. (Don't assume that your plan disallows it without checking!)

Ideally, your doctor's participation should begin with the onset of symptoms, especially with early, subtle, or intermittent symptoms. As I have explained, calling your doctor immediately will yield the dividend of knowing whether you need to go to the ER and what form of transportation he or she would prefer you to use.

It is especially helpful for your doctor to call the ER to alert the staff of your arrival and to give them your health information. Ideally, your doctor will join you soon at the ER, perhaps even meeting you there on your arrival. Your doctor should participate to the greatest extent feasible in selecting one of the treatment options presented in the previous chapter. People prefer to be treated in hospitals as close as possible to their own homes and by their own doctors. This continuing process should begin in the ER.

Currently, far too little is being said about the once prominent topic of easing emotional stress during a heart attack. Increasing emotional stress at this time can have very serious consequences, including causing heart discomfort to worsen or recur. It can even cause heart rhythm irregularities that are potentially lethal. I have already noted the possibly detrimental effects of sirens and rapid speed during ambulance transportation; it is possible that the extremely low frequency of adverse events seen in patients traveling by car is due to car travel being less emotionally stressful. Your doctor's presence is even more vital in alleviating nervous tension, particularly the very frequent fear of death. By no means am I the first to become aware of this, but it has been my pleasure and privilege to immediately see the spirits of hundreds of my patients brighten on my arrival—which tells me how helpful the familiar face of a doctor can be.

I am dwelling on this because in recent medical publications I have not seen the barest mention by a high-level authority of the value of your physician in heart care. It is my hope that one effect of this book will be to bring about a reawakening of interest in this topic. In some quarters, particularly in managed care situations, your doctor is called the "primary physician" or the "primary care provider." On the other hand, patients usually refer to their personal physician as "my doctor" and say it with pride. The pride doctors feel about their relationship with their patients was clearly illustrated by the extensive interviews of internists and family practitioners reported by the REACT designers referred to earlier. In your own case, ensuring a productive long-term relationship with your physician requires some thought and effort on your part.

Tips for Engaging a Personal Doctor

Your personal physician will most likely be a family practitioner or internist. Today's cardiologists are almost entirely occupied with catheterization laboratory and other high-technology services and in-hospital patient care. Consequently, they function almost exclusively as consultants to your personal physician in heart attacks, returning you to your own doctor after the special need ends.

If you belong to a managed care organization that permits you to call a personal physician in case of an emergency and you do not yet have a personal physician, your first step is to call the managed care office to see which physicians are available near your home. Next, find out what their credentials are (particularly whether they are board certified), how they are paid, and whether, if you so choose, you can change doctors without leaving the system.

If you do not belong to a managed care association but have health insurance that covers personal physician involvement in emergencies and do not yet have a personal physician, inquire among your friends about their doctors and their experiences with them. If this does not yield a likely match, consult your local medical society or the hospital of your choice, both of which will have referral services.

Whether you have managed care or not, call for an appointment and state that your purpose is deciding whether you wish to become a patient. If that request is denied, make another choice. If that request is granted, it probably means that the doctor is interested in having you as a patient, a very important point.

At this conference, you need to ask the doctor the following questions:

1. Do you do complete physical examinations head-to-toe on the first visit and at least on an annual basis thereafter, with me unclothed to ensure a comprehensive exam?
2. Are you willing to see me as often as needed on a year-round basis, including about issues of blood pressure, cholesterol, and weight control?
3. Will you obtain ECGs, chest X-rays, and blood tests such as cholesterol measurements as often as needed?
4. Will you spend time on office visits advising me about prevention of heart disease and strokes?
5. Will you advise me about how to attend to possible heart attacks and strokes, and in such an event, do you wish to be called, or should I rely entirely on 911?
6. If you do wish to be called, how do I reach you or your alternate immediately day or night?
7. If I wind up in the emergency room with a possible heart attack or stroke, will you come to see me?
8. If I call for you at your office about a question that is important to me, can I speak directly with you, or would I be allowed only to talk with your nurse?

Think of these requests as the *patient's bill of rights.* If the response to even one of these requests is negative, consider seeking another physician. Most doctors respect patients who show commitment to their health care, so do not hesitate to ask these questions. It also helps to take a list of your questions with you when you have your office visits, since this usually yields more information in the time available.

Remember, if your doctor is not available, or if your health plan does not allow you to contact your personal physician in a heart emergency, get to the hospital by the quickest, most appropriate means possible. If your health coverage does not permit your personal physician to be available in emergencies, use your next appointment as an opportunity to ask what he or she recommends regarding transportation and selection of emergency rooms (if more than one is close by) in the event of your experiencing any of the early warning signs when you are at or near home. That way you are getting your doctor's advice in advance—and it will help you to formulate a plan in case of an emergency.

Part II

How a Heart Attack Is Treated

Chapter 7

Thrombolysis

The Heart Attack Treatment Breakthrough

In 1979, Dr. Peter Rentrop was the first in the world to carry out thrombolysis, the breakthrough treatment that dissolves the blood clot in a coronary artery that causes a heart attack.[1] Rentrop did this by injecting the drug streptokinase directly into the artery through a slender tube, or catheter, after the clot's location had been determined by the catheterization laboratory examination known as coronary angiography (see Chapter 8). Partly through the advocacy of Dr. William Ganz of Cedars of Lebanon Hospital in Los Angeles, thrombolysis was rapidly taken up by cardiologists across the country, but its use was limited by the necessity of its being carried out in cath labs, available in only a small minority of hospitals.

In the early 1980s, the Italian GISSI Group, an association of scores of hospitals, demonstrated the effectiveness of giving streptokinase by intravenous injection, making it feasible to administer thrombolysis in hospitals without cath labs. In 1986, GISSI reported studies of thousands of patients showing that if this treatment was given during the first sixty minutes of symptoms, deaths were reduced by 49 percent, and if given before the end of the third hour symptoms, were reduced by 25 percent.[2]

As I mentioned previously, this data led me to call the first sixty minutes of symptoms the golden hour for treating heart attacks, a term now widely used in the field. (I borrowed the term from trauma care, where it was used in reference to highway trauma victims whose deaths were cut in half if they were gotten into operating rooms within sixty minutes of the injury.)

Not only do GISSI's positive results still stand, but Dr. W. Douglas Weaver, Henry Ford Hospital's division head of cardiovascular medicine, recently reported a study showing that 30 percent of patients receiving thrombolysis within the first hour showed *no* evidence of damage to the heart—"It wasn't there!" Weaver exclaimed.[3] In Chapter 2, I also mentioned the earlier report that thrombolysis during the first seventy minutes of symptoms cut the death rate to 1.2 percent.[4] Since the primary purpose of this book is to educate you in order to prevent needless heart damage, I am devoting this chapter to amplifying the vital subject of thrombolysis.

On November 13, 1987, the pharmaceutical firm Genentech Laboratories introduced a different type of thrombolytic agent, the tissue plasminogen activator (TPA) class of drugs. Tests involving thousands of patients showed these drugs to be somewhat superior to streptokinase in that they are more effective in opening obstructed arteries.[5] Since then, additional TPA drugs have become available. These drugs are usually given intravenously in a single injection over a period of a few seconds, replacing the previous prolonged injection, making the treatment very convenient.

These "clot-buster" drugs that can stop a heart attack "in its tracks" can be injected into the vein within fifteen to thirty minutes of arrival in the emergency room (figs. 7.1–7.2). I noted earlier the enormous value of this treatment during the first three hours of symptoms, but research shows there may be some benefit between three and six hours, or even between six and twelve hours, although the benefit at these later times is limited.

One large study showed that in patients receiving thrombolysis within the first two hours of symptoms, the death rate was less than half that of patients whose symptoms had begun six hours before.[6] The sharp reduction in treatment benefits at three hours is due to the fact that the death of heart muscle after a heart attack is usually complete by three hours after the beginning of symptoms. This means that after three hours, there is little if any heart muscle left to salvage. Early treatment is enormously beneficial precisely because it saves heart muscle. The aging of blood clots in coronary arteries that cause

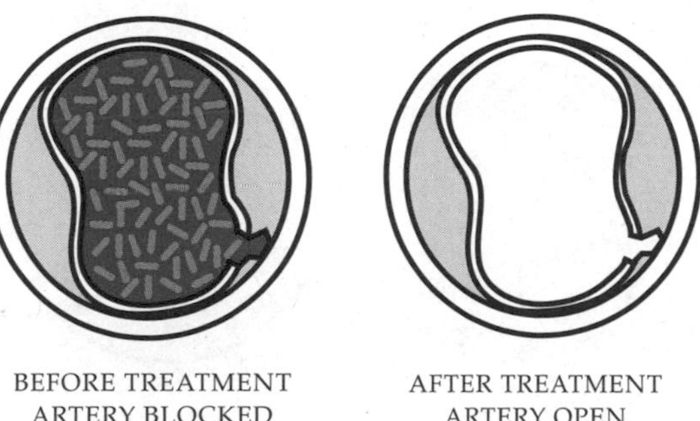

Fig. 7.1 "CLOT-BUSTER" THROMBOLYSIS

Blood clot–dissolving heart attack treatment eliminates excessive clot formed to seal cracks in cholesterol deposits. Artery pulsation during heartbeats causes such cracking. Restoring blood flow to the heart downstream within three hours has been shown to reduce death by 25 percent. Thrombolysis also benefits persons with strokes caused by clots.

heart attacks makes it progressively more difficult to dissolve them by thrombolysis, a factor adding to the need for early treatment.

A small minority of patients are not eligible for thrombolysis treatment. This includes those individuals with recent surgery or bodily injury that might cause bleeding during treatment, those with a recent stroke or stomach or duodenal ulcers with recent hemorrhage, and those with hypertension (high blood pressure), unless the hypertension can be reduced promptly with treatment.

The only important possible complication from thrombolysis is if it causes bleeding, chiefly a hemorrhagic stroke (see Chapter 20). The risk of stroke from thrombolysis is very small, and is only a very small fraction of the risk of having an untreated heart attack. If you are eligible for thrombolysis, this risk should not deter you from receiving the treatment.

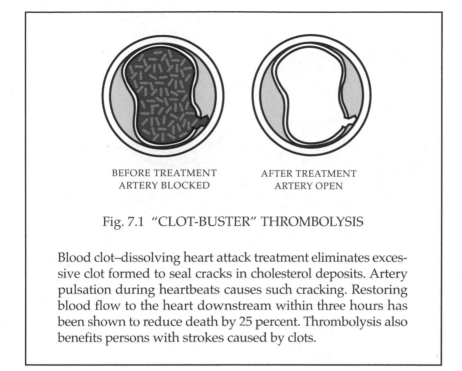

Emergency room physicians are highly skilled at administering thrombolysis treatment. Although the presence of your personal

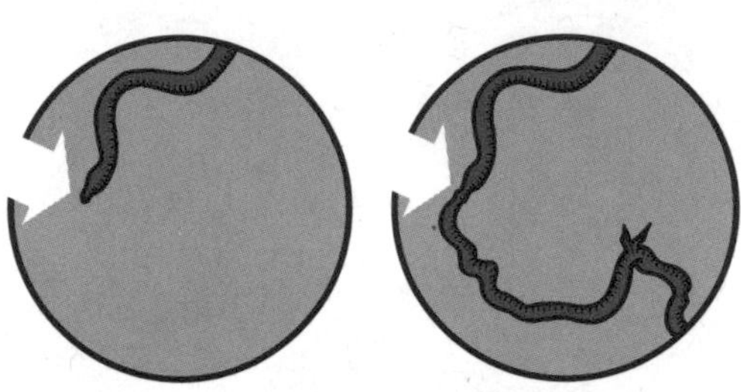

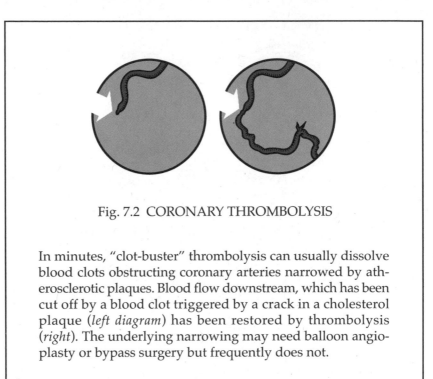

Fig. 7.2 CORONARY THROMBOLYSIS

In minutes, "clot-buster" thrombolysis can usually dissolve blood clots obstructing coronary arteries narrowed by atherosclerotic plaques. Blood flow downstream, which has been cut off by a blood clot triggered by a crack in a cholesterol plaque (*left diagram*) has been restored by thrombolysis (*right*). The underlying narrowing may need balloon angioplasty or bypass surgery but frequently does not.

physician in the ER while you are there is beneficial, it is not necessary or desirable to delay thrombolysis until your doctor arrives.

Where should thrombolysis treatment be carried out? As I have said, the answer is simple: at the hospital nearest you, whether it is a small community hospital or a larger facility. Everywhere in the United States you are only minutes away from this type of treatment. Your only chance of getting this treatment during the golden hour is by recognizing your symptoms promptly and going by car to your nearest emergency room. That is why I am repeating it once again: the most important word in getting lifesaving treatment in a heart emergency is *early*—early recognition and early treatment.

In the United States there have been a number of programs in which paramedics administer thrombolysis before hospital arrival in order to start treatment earlier, but this practice has not been widely adopted. In Chapter 5, I mentioned Weaver's comment about the "fragmented" EMS system in our country. Weaver further states that the system of administering thrombolysis by EMS teams is more successful in Europe, where physicians staff the ambulances. For a paramedic to start thrombolysis treatment for a patient before hospital arrival requires several steps. First, the paramedic must record an ECG in the patient's home. Then, since it is unlikely for a paramedic to start thrombolysis in a moving ambulance, the paramedic must transmit the ECG to the ER physician for a decision whether to treat, and then the paramedic must receive orders. This takes time. Next, if told to proceed with thrombolysis on site, the paramedic must establish a satisfactory intravenous line, which may be very awkward under less than ideal light in the patient's home. My opinion is that from the time you decide to seek help, thrombolysis treatment can be under way more quickly by more expert hands in more ideal circumstances than by ambulance staffs, notwithstanding their high levels of training.

The response to thrombolysis treatment can usually be ascertained by closely observing repeated ECGs (fig. 7.3). If thrombolysis is successful, the medications to reduce repeat blood clotting listed in the previous chapter will be used. If thrombolysis treatment fails, which does not often happen during the golden hour, it may be decided to take you to a cath lab in the same or another hospital for the procedure referred to as "rescue" angioplasty. At this point, you would probably be beyond the time at which heart muscle can be salvaged. But remember, just because heart muscle has died in the area of the heart that has been cut off from blood does not mean you will die. The heart can lose about 40 percent of the muscle and remain able to function, although to a more limited extent, which will require medication or other treatment.

If rescue angioplasty is elected following thrombolysis (see Chapter 9), there is a debate about whether it should be done immediately or at a later time. Your doctor can help you decide whether to accept or reject the recommendation of rescue angioplasty and when it should be performed.

Witnessing and experiencing the successful interruption of a heart attack with thrombolysis can be a wonderful experience for patient, family, and doctor. When I had the privilege of treating the first patient at St. John's to receive thrombolysis, I was able to get a TPA flowing into his veins within twenty minutes of his arrival and within

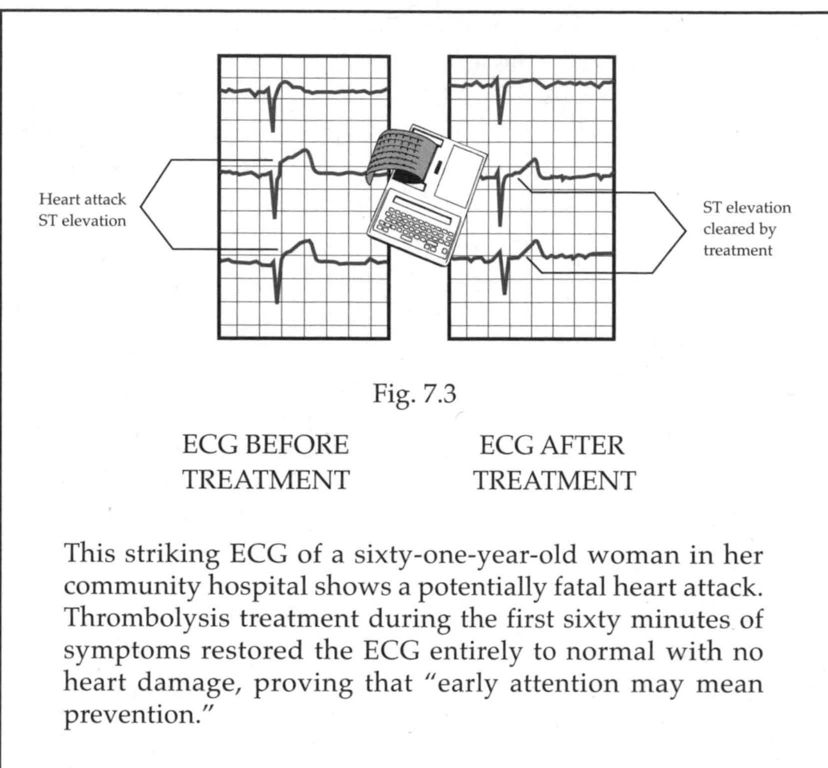

Fig. 7.3

ECG BEFORE TREATMENT

ECG AFTER TREATMENT

This striking ECG of a sixty-one-year-old woman in her community hospital shows a potentially fatal heart attack. Thrombolysis treatment during the first sixty minutes of symptoms restored the ECG entirely to normal with no heart damage, proving that "early attention may mean prevention."

sixty minutes from the onset of his symptoms. (His pain had been relieved with intravenous morphine immediately on his admission.) A series of ECGs showed complete clearing of signs of his heart attack before completion of the ninety-minute treatment. The patient, all smiles, shook my hand in appreciation. Blood tests showed no heart damage. It was a thrilling, miraculous event!

CHAPTER 8

Coronary Angiograms

What Are They and What Do They Accomplish?

Throughout most of medical history, doctors were able to study diseased coronary arteries only after a patient's death, but in 1960 Dr. Mason Sones of the Cleveland Clinic in Ohio discovered the process of coronary angiography, a method of photographing these arteries during life.[1] The ability to obtain these photographs, known as coronary angiograms, opened up a new era in the understanding and treatment of coronary heart diseases (CHD).

The year 1960 also witnessed the bringing together in Springfield of three other historic advances: electrical defibrillation of a fatal heart rhythm in order to restore normal heart rhythm, closed-chest cardiac massage to sustain circulation during cardiopulmonary resuscitation, and the establishment at St. John's Hospital of the nation's first cardiovascular care unit to group heart disease patients to better carry out these lifesaving procedures. The key to applying these new advances was the wealth of information about the arteries of the heart that was provided by Sones's discovery.

Coronary angiography begins with cardiac catheterization. There are two cardiac catheterization procedures. The first, and by far the most frequent, combines what is known as left-heart catheterization with coronary angiography. The other, right-heart catheterization, is an entirely separate procedure that is usually related to disease involving lung circulation and the heart's right ventricle. In left-heart catheterization, after deadening the skin to make the procedure painless, a very slender tube, or catheter, is inserted into an artery at the groin or in the arm, then passed through the aorta to the top of the heart (fig. 8.1). There, the catheter is inserted into the interior of the left ventricle, which is why the procedure is called left-heart catheterization. This permits study of the function of the heart muscle and of the aortic and mitral valves.

After dye has been injected to provide photographic contrast, motion picture photographs at thirty frames per second record the action of the heart during the procedure. The coronary angiography is done by inserting another catheter sequentially into the mouths of the right and left coronary arteries at the base of the aorta, at its point of origin. Dye is injected, and its flow through the artery is recorded by the camera. While this is taking place, the cardiologist observes it on a high-magnification screen. Multiple angles of photography record all profiles of the artery. The flow of the dye can be followed through the small artery branches and into the heart muscle. This gives very important information about interference with blood flow at any point in the circuit of arteries. All obstructions but the very slightest can be detected during the examination. Minutes later, the cardiologist can study the 35mm-film frames in detail.

It is difficult to describe the audience's excitement at Sones's presentation of his discovery at the 1960 annual meeting of the American Heart Association. It revolutionized the treatment of patients with heart disease. Of the vast amount of new information about coronary heart disease provided by coronary angiography, two discoveries were especially important. First, coronary angiography disproved the previous conclusion that blood clots found in coronary arteries after death from a heart attack formed after death. Instead, it was found by examinations during life that the blood clots were the *cause* of heart attacks. This opened up a whole new era of research to find out how to deal with these clots. Second, coronary angiography led to the discovery that most heart attacks do *not* result from the complete obstruction of severely narrowed arteries; rather, they occur during the early stages of cholesterol deposition, when the plaques are thinner and more likely to crack or rupture. These ruptures lead to the blood clot that causes the obstruction and resulting heart attack. This new understanding explains why so few patients experi-

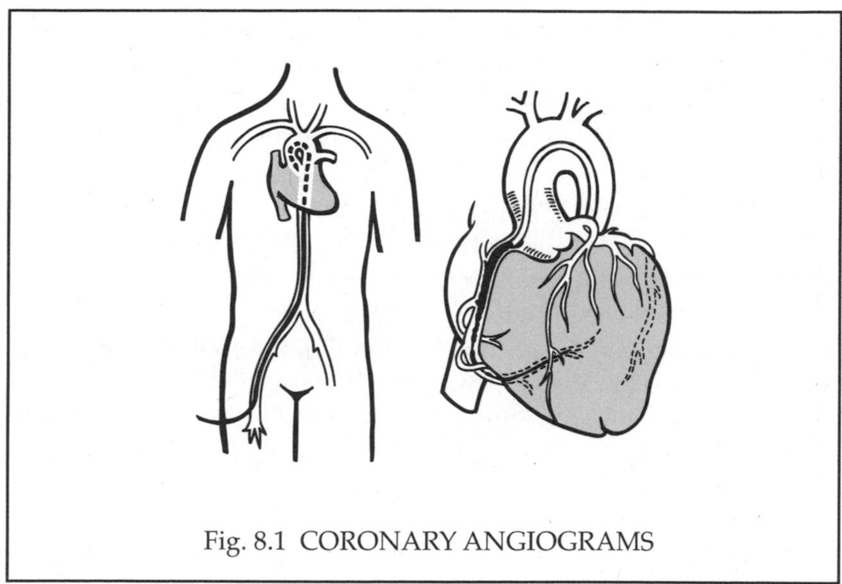

Fig. 8.1 CORONARY ANGIOGRAMS

encing heart attacks have forewarning periods of angina on physical exertion. It is because the large majority of heart attack sufferers are not forewarned by angina that it is so crucial to recognize the very earliest symptoms of a heart attack when they do occur.

Although the decades-long practice of photographically portraying coronary artery narrowings remains the gold standard in deciding the need for bypass surgery, there have been notable advances in more accurately studying coronary artery narrowings. Digital photography has replaced some of the previous "film units." Since the photographic process provides only profile views of cholesterol deposits without giving information about the characteristics of the plaque related to the risk of cracking, intravascular ultrasound (IVUS) catheters have been developed to fill in this gap. IVUS catheters have a tiny ultrasound sensor at the tip that provides remarkable information about the full circumference and content of the plaque and the risk it poses. Other advances include rapid computerized tomography (CT) scanning.

The original CT equipment showed images of thin "slices" of body tissues. To give greater breadth of images, multiple-slice equipment was developed, leading to the present sixty-four-slice model. As cholesterol plaques age and thicken, calcium deposits increase. This advanced CT examination measures the amount and extent of calcium deposits. The quantity of calcium thus disclosed is expressed as the "calcium score," reflecting the severity of the atherosclerosis.

An intravenous injection of dye gives information about a short segment of the channel through the artery. Magnetic resonance imaging (MRI) also gives information, but neither of these examinations yields the detailed information about the entirety of the coronary artery system that is provided by coronary angiography, and neither is usually involved in the treatment of an acute heart attack. Several other highly technical examinations are useful in diagnosing coronary heart disease but are also not usually a part of acute heart attack care. Among these are exercise and chemical stress testing, ultrasound examination (echocardiography), and a number of nuclear and electrophysiological studies. Describing these complex procedures is beyond the scope of this book, which is focused on acute heart care, nor is it feasible to summarize here the excellent methods of diagnosing and treating other major disorders such as congestive heart failure and peripheral vascular disease (atherosclerotic and other involvements of the arteries and veins of the abdomen and legs). Coronary angiography, however, is used extensively in the investigation and management of acute heart attacks in association with balloon coronary angioplasty, the subject of the next chapter.

As mentioned, of the 4,942 acute-care hospitals in the United States, fewer than one-third have the cardiac catheterization laboratories necessary to do coronary angiograms, but that number is increasing. The decision to conduct coronary angiography is made on consultation with a cardiologist who will take into consideration a broad range of possible heart disease conditions and will use the examination to help decide about treatment. Coronary angiography is an extremely common procedure. If your personal physician is part of your emergency heart care, it is likely that he or she will participate in whatever decision is reached about conducting the examination.

Chapter 9

Balloon Coronary Angioplasty

What It Accomplishes, What It Does Not Accomplish, and How This Affects Your Choices about Treatment

The narrowing of an artery by cholesterol deposits is the condition known as atherosclerosis. Dr. Andreas Gruentzig of Switzerland performed the first balloon angioplasty of a coronary artery in 1977 in order to widen the narrowed artery.[1] Gruentzig had worked extensively with engineers to develop a slender balloon that expanded evenly through its length rather than in a ball to widen the artery. The procedure Gruentzig perfected remains the standard today. It is carried out in the cardiac catheterization laboratory after coronary angiography has disclosed one or more cholesterol deposits large enough to interfere with blood flow through an artery. These deposits are usually localized and soft enough to be compressed, which will open the artery for blood flow. If the angiography examination reveals these deposits, the angioplasty procedure is usually carried out in the same session.

This procedure involves inserting a catheter with a slender deflated balloon at the tip through an artery in the groin or in the arm and passing the balloon-tipped catheter through the aorta to the opening of the artery that is to be dilated. Over a guiding wire, the balloon is centered in the obstructed area. When this is accomplished, the balloon is repeatedly inflated under high pressure for sixty to ninety seconds each time until the desired result is achieved. Arteries that have been narrowed up to 95 percent can usually be reduced to 10 to 30 percent narrowing, restoring flow practically to normal (fig. 9.1). Narrowings in two or all three major vessels may be dilated during the same session.

The American Heart Association reported in 2007 that 1,285,000 of these procedures were carried out in 2004 in the United States.[2] The most frequent use of balloon angioplasty is to reduce arterial narrowings from cholesterol deposits in patients who have severely narrowed arteries but who have not experienced a heart attack. Recently, balloon coronary angioplasty is very much in the medical and public news. In this chapter, I shall give you an overview of this very important topic.

This procedure has three principal uses: to relieve chronic angina by dilating coronary narrowings that interfere with blood flow during exercise or stress, to relieve acutely worsened (unstable) angina that might otherwise result in a heart attack, and to treat heart attacks after they occur. When Gruentzig introduced angioplasty in 1977, it had already been learned that most heart attacks resulted from cracking or rupture of the caps of thinner cholesterol deposits, and the use of Gruentzig's procedure to widen arterial channels by compressing thicker cholesterol deposits soon showed that the procedure did not reduce heart attacks. It was promptly adopted for the relief of angina, for which it was immediately effective. During the thirty years of its use, the frequency of carrying out the procedure to relieve angina steadily increased. It is now estimated that 85 percent of the more than 1 million coronary angioplasties being done each year are for chronic or stable angina.[3] It also came to be used in some cases of more severe angina as an alternative to coronary artery bypass surgery.

Meanwhile, medical (that is, nonprocedural) treatment of angina was improving substantially. This consisted of developing better medications for the prevention and relief of episodes of anginal discomfort and a reduction in coronary heart disease risks, particularly cholesterol and triglyceride abnormality, high blood pressure, smoking, weight excess, and physical inactivity. Carrying out all these measures came to be known as "optimal medical therapy." When the success of this therapy became apparent, the American College of Cardiology (ACC) and the American Heart Association established guidelines for angina treatment that specified that optimal medical therapy be the

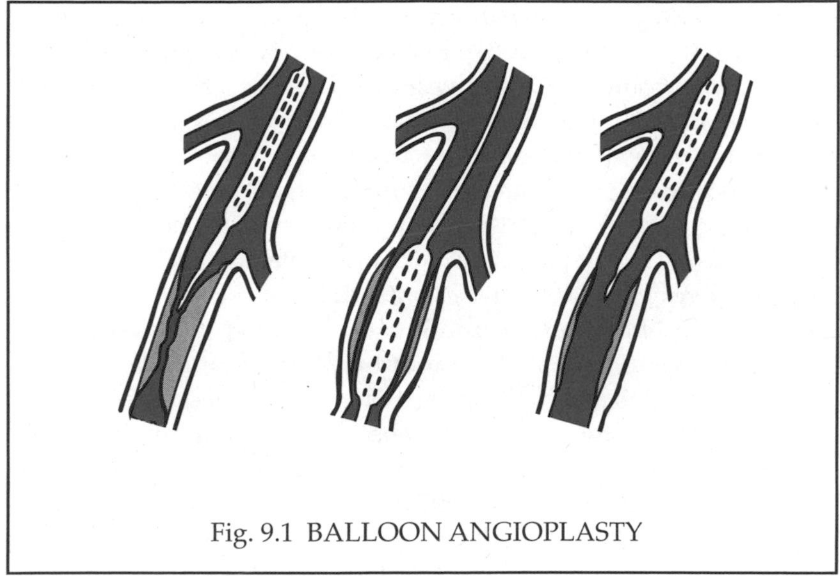

Fig. 9.1 BALLOON ANGIOPLASTY

initial treatment for chronic stable angina, reserving angioplasty for treatment failures. However, many cardiologists did not follow this recommendation, continuing to use angioplasty as their initial treatment of angina, leading to the million or so annual procedures.

Some authorities became concerned about so many cardiologists failing to follow the AHA/ACC guidelines and conducted a number of small studies that showed no benefit of angioplasty over optimal medical therapy. To further resolve this issue, a large study was started in 1999 in fifty hospitals in the United States and Canada to compare the results of the two types of treatment in consecutive patients over a period averaging 4.6 years. Two groups of patients were given carefully administered optimal medical therapy. Angioplasty was added as treatment for one of the groups. The results were reported in March 2007.[4] They showed that adding angioplasty to optimal medical therapy did not reduce heart attacks, deaths, repeat hospital admissions, bypass surgery, or strokes. Angioplasty reduced angina severity at first, but angina severity in the two groups later equalized. This report made news-media headlines nationwide. A later report on the comparative costs of the two types of treatment and one on quality-of-life assessments were promised. One national news service made a statement that balloon coronary angioplasties cost an average of forty thousand dollars.[5] (See my remarks later in this chapter about costs in Springfield.) There can be no doubt that cardiologists and hospitals have a huge financial incentive to opt for adding angioplasty to medical treatment. It is uncertain how much effect this information will have on future treatment choices and on insurance coverage. Some patients or their insurance carriers or both may be willing to pay the extra cost of angioplasty to obtain this temporary betterment of anginal discomfort. From the first, balloon angioplasty has been an alternative to coronary bypass surgery (installing a vein or artery graft to provide a detour around the obstruction) for patients with atherosclerotic arteries. The decision about which procedure to use must be made on an individual basis.

Today, the most frequent complication of angioplasty, restenosis (the process of scar-tissue formation resulting from balloon injury to the artery wall), has largely been solved. In the past, restenosis advanced sufficiently in 30 to 40 percent of cases to require repeat angioplasty, or sometimes bypass surgery, within six months of the first procedure. The solution was the introduction of stents, wire-mesh expandable tubes that are inserted after the balloon is removed and then expanded to the full diameter of the vessel, stabilizing the injured artery wall (fig. 9.2).[6] The initial "bare-metal" version of the stent reduced restenosis to about 20 percent. Very infrequently, inflating the balloon may cause a tear in the wall of the artery, a problem that stents also reduced by providing scaffolding for injured artery walls, making emergency bypass surgery to deal with artery tears necessary in only a minority of cases. As a result, numerous hospitals with cath labs but no emergency heart surgery capability now have balloon angioplasty programs.

The years 2003 and 2004 saw the introduction of the drug-eluting stent. In this procedure, drugs that hamper the development of scar tissue are impregnated into materials used to coat bare-metal stents. These drugs are then released (eluted) over a period of weeks into the surrounding artery wall, greatly reducing the proliferation of scar tissue. Patients often require two or more of these stents. They are more expensive than the bare-metal version, but in many hospitals drug-eluting stents have largely replaced the bare-metal variety.

Within a year after their introduction, however, it was clear that although the reduction of restenosis was near complete, there was a

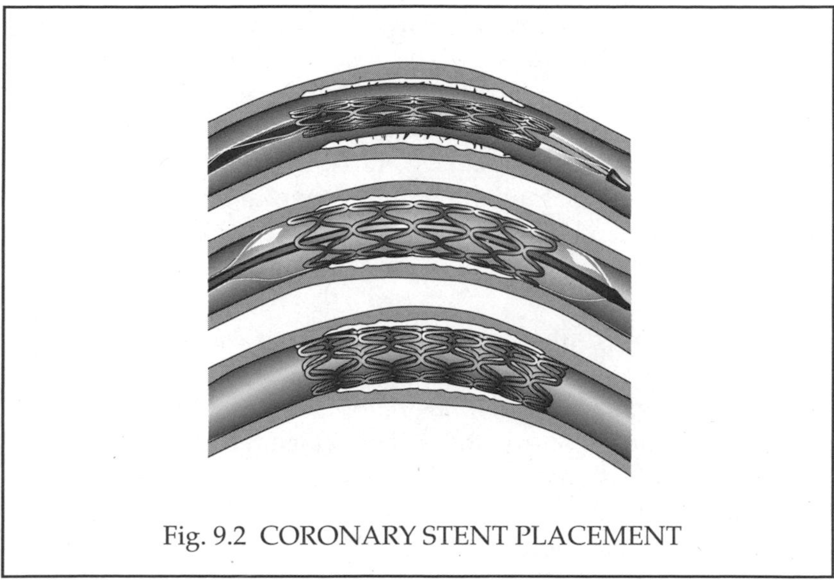

Fig. 9.2 CORONARY STENT PLACEMENT

later complication: the abrupt obstruction of the artery by a blood clot, causing a heart attack, sometimes fatal.[7] Although some say the risk of complications from drug-eluting stents is outweighed by their benefits, there is consensus that a solution must be found, and a great deal of work is being done to find one. Approaches include being more selective about which patients are given drug-eluting stents, longer-term use of anti-blood-clotting medications such as clopidogril (Plavix) with drug-eluting stents, use of a different drug coating for the stents, and use of different materials in constructing the stent coils.

Sometimes, in conjunction with angioplasty or separately, a device is used to actually remove cholesterol plaque from the artery wall. This device is a rapidly rotating mechanism at the end of the catheter that shaves or abrades the plaque, collecting the fragments for removal.

Another method of reducing the frequency of restenosis is brachytherapy, a treatment in which a catheter tipped with radioactive material is inserted into the angioplasty site for a few minutes after removal of the balloon. This irradiation hinders the development of scar tissue in the artery wall. The technical requirements of brachytherapy limit the number of hospitals able to provide it.

Coronary Angioplasty for the Treatment of Unstable Angina

It is coming to be a frequent practice to do coronary angiography when angina worsens (becomes unstable) to determine whether there is an artery narrowing that seems likely to close completely and cause a heart attack. In this situation, angioplasty may avert that event. Anti-blood-clotting and other drugs are intensively used in such cases.

Coronary Angioplasty in Heart Attack Treatment

The widespread use of balloon angioplasty in treating atherosclerotic coronary artery narrowings set the stage for many in the early 1980s to adopt this procedure for reopening the channel in arteries obstructed by blood clots in acute heart attacks. Many of you may be abruptly and unexpectedly confronted by the necessity of deciding whether a heart attack will be treated with thrombolysis or by balloon angioplasty. Learning how to make the best decision before the need arises is the next step in your heart care education.

As you know, in the event of a heart attack, the length of time from the onset of symptoms to the start of treatment determines your odds of survival and the likely degree of impairment in your later ability to function. Both are greatly enhanced by getting treatment before the end of the third hour of symptoms when death of muscle in the blocked area of the heart is complete. The first portion of the time of symptom onset to treatment is the period before hospital arrival, which Dr. Eric J. Topol, the chief academic officer and Scripps health and senior consultant of the Division of Cardiovascular Diseases at the Scripps Research Institute in La Jolla, California, has defined the median in the United States as 2.7 hours. Since this median means that as many patients arrive before 2.7 hours as after, perhaps half of our country's heart attack patients are arriving at the hospital within the three-hour window when treatment is most beneficial. I can virtually guarantee all readers who learn the information in this book that in the event of a heart attack, the number of you who will get to the hospital during the first, second, and third hours of symptoms will exceed the present averages. If you learn and respond promptly to the early warning signs, you will have a good measure of control of the time factor of symptom onset to treatment.

The remainder of the symptom-onset-to-treatment time is the time spent after arrival at the emergency room. If thrombolysis treatment is chosen, the interval to starting it is known as door-to-needle time. The American Heart Association and American College of Cardiology guidelines call for this time to be 30 minutes or less.[8] This goal is usually achieved, a reduction from the previous national average of 60 minutes. Some unofficially advocate a door-to-needle time of 15 minutes.[9]

The time from arrival to insertion of the balloon into the artery in the cath lab is known as door-to-balloon time. The AHA / ACC guidelines call for door-to-balloon time not to exceed 90 minutes and not to be longer than 60 minutes after suitability for thrombolysis has been determined.[10] Dr. Cindy Grines of William Beaumont Hospital in Royal Oak, Michigan—one of the leading proponents of angioplasty for all heart attack patients—recently stated that the door-to-balloon time in her hospital is 120 minutes, but she states that benefits still result from angioplasty after the 120-minute delay, and she feels the 90-minute rule is too strict.[11] Others, however, continue to emphasize the necessity of a shorter time frame. A number of reports show the importance of doing angioplasty as early as possible.[12] The findings of one recent study support the AHA / ACC guidelines of a 90-minute door-to-balloon cutoff time for treatment in order to optimize possible benefits.[13]

Several factors may increase the door-to-balloon time. One of the most common is the time required to assemble the cath lab staff and the physician operator. This may take time even during the day, but it is especially true at night; few hospitals can maintain staff on the premises at night. Some hospitals perform angioplasty only during the day, using thrombolysis at night. At any hour, the cath lab equipment and staff may be involved in a procedure that cannot be interrupted when a decision is made to treat a newly arrived heart attack patient, and this may cause a further delay.

With the above information in mind, how does the time to treatment for thrombolysis compare to that of balloon angioplasty? For thrombolysis patients, if you add the U.S. median hospital arrival time of 2.7 hours to the current uniformly achieved 30-minute door-to-needle time, the result is a symptom-onset-to-needle time of 3 hours and 12 minutes. Since, as noted earlier, a great many patients arrive in less than 2.7 hours, adding the 30-minute door-to-needle time means that many arrive during the 3-hour period when deaths can be reduced by 25 to 49 percent.

It is clear that the symptom-onset-to-treatment time when angioplasty is performed is far longer than the time required if thrombolysis is chosen. Adding the 120-minute door-to-balloon time reported by Grines in her hospital to the national average of 2.7 hours of prehospital time gives a total of 4 hours and 42 minutes. This is far in excess of the 3-hour window for optimal treatment. Even if patients arrive in less than 2.7 hours—say, 90 minutes from symptom onset—the time of symptom onset to balloon insertion is well over 3 hours. Later, I will discuss the issue of a further increase in time if the receiving hospital does not have a cath lab and a patient is transported to a cath lab hospital for balloon angioplasty.

How do the results of thrombolysis and angioplasty compare? If, like a majority of patients, you are eligible for thrombolysis and get to the hospital in time for it to be administered during the first, second, or third hour of symptoms, angioplasty falls far short of this treatment. Remember, thrombolysis cuts the number of deaths in half if given in the first hour and by 25 percent if given before the end of the third hour. The difference in results from thrombolysis versus angioplasty is due to the very long door-to-balloon time for angioplasty. Topol emphasizes this difference by saying that angioplasty is satisfactory treatment "if you have your MI [heart attack] at the door of the cath lab."[14]

In Chapter 7, I quoted Weaver's report showing that, in patients receiving thrombolysis during the first hour, 30 percent showed no evidence of heart damage. Weaver went on to explain that "in patients who present very early, thrombolysis looks very good, because in patients who present early and go to the cath lab, there is no early—it is just impossible. When you get to the hospital and to the cath lab you are out of that window, and that's what makes thrombolysis look particularly good early." I also mentioned that the GISSI Group studies documented the excellent benefits from thrombolysis through the third hour.

Two studies throw important light on this subject. The first, done at the Mayo Clinic in Rochester, Minnesota, used very sophisticated nuclear imaging equipment to measure the extent of heart muscle deprived of blood by the obstructed blood vessel in the heart attack. This rapid examination was performed on the patients' arrival, followed by assigning some of them to thrombolysis and others to angioplasty. The examination was repeated after treatment, at hospital discharge. Comparing the results of the two examinations showed how much muscle was saved by treatment. Data from those who received treatment during the first two hours of symptoms were compared with data from patients who received treatment after two hours of symptoms. Those patients who received treatment by either method during the first two hours of symptoms had major or near-complete salvage of the affected muscle, whereas those treated after two hours had very little salvage unless the affected muscle had received blood from a dual or collateral blood supply beyond the point of artery obstruction (a structural element of the heart that varies from person to person). One in three of the patients treated with thrombolysis received it during the first two hours, whereas only one in eleven angioplasty patients was treated during the first two hours because of the long door-to-balloon time, due to the lack of available operating rooms or staff or other circumstances. This means that the opportunity for major muscle salvage is very infrequent with angioplasty.[15]

The second study was reported at the November 2006 annual meeting of the American Heart Association. The report stated that in hospitals carrying out angioplasty for heart attack patients, only 30 percent had door-to-balloon times of the prescribed 90 minutes or less.[16] Thus, 70 percent of the patients in this large study did not receive angioplasty during the period in which the American Heart Association and American College of Cardiology declare it to be beneficial and appropriate. And remember, this study just accounted for door-to-balloon time once the patients arrived at the emergency room. To calculate the total time until angioplasty is performed, we have to add the time it takes to respond to symptoms and get to the hospital.

What are the results in patients arriving after three hours of symptoms? Since heart muscle death in the affected area is usually considered complete by three hours after the onset of the attack, there is little if any muscle to preserve in that area. This means that the benefits of any treatment at this point are limited in terms of that specific muscle. The Mayo Clinic's Dr. Bernard Gersh recently stated that when patients arrive for treatment "three hours out from the onset of symptoms . . . it is too late to make a difference."[17] Although this is largely true in terms of treating muscle that has been lost, treatment for a heart attack after three hours is still very important and is often lifesaving in reducing complications from the heart attack. Once patients are in the hospital, heart rhythms can be monitored and controlled and congestive heart failure can be attended to.

There is, however, controversy surrounding treatment options for the heart attack itself after three hours. Because blood clots causing heart attacks become more difficult to dissolve as they grow older, an obstructed artery can be reopened more completely after three hours by angioplasty than by thrombolysis. Initially, this led to great emphasis on the "open artery" value of angioplasty for heart attacks. Proponents started to declare a policy of angioplasty for all patients with acute heart attacks. However, it was ultimately found that when angioplasty reopened a major coronary artery channel that had been obstructed by the blood clot causing the attack, in half the cases the blood flowing through the reopened artery did not reach the heart muscle downstream, and in all other cases restoration of flow was not complete.

It was assumed at first that blood-clot fragments released by balloon compression were obstructing branches of the major artery as the clot fragments flowed downstream. But since a number of devices designed to trap these fragments during the angioplasty procedure did not improve blood flow to the injured heart muscle, it is now thought that the impaired downstream blood flow is caused by injury to blood vessels during the period when they are deprived of nourishing blood flow.[18]

Today, some specialists say that as a treatment for heart attacks, the primary benefit from angioplasty's ability to dilate artery narrowings is a reduction in short- and long-term complications from an attack rather than improving survival from the acute heart attack itself.[19] However, this claim has been called into question by a very large study of Medicare patients that showed that the five-year survival rate after treatment for heart attacks in communities where angioplasty was the predominant treatment was little or no better than in those communities where angioplasty was used infrequently.[20] Thus, angioplasty's ability to reduce long-term complications and risks after a heart attack is as yet unproven and must be further researched.

One aspect of delaying angioplasty beyond the recommended ninety minutes was reported at the 2006 AHA meeting mentioned earlier. For various reasons, it is a frequent practice for some cardiologists to perform angioplasty for a heart attack days after the episode. The study reported no long-term benefit from angioplasty performed three days or later after a heart attack and noted that this delayed treatment was possibly harmful, since subsequent deaths of patients with angioplasty were 17 percent compared with 15 percent without it. It was speculated that discontinuing these late angioplasties would reduce the number of these procedures in the United States by one hundred thousand annually.[21] This would produce a great savings for patients and insurers, since the cost of angioplasty is far greater than that of thrombolysis.[22] I believe it is inevitable that the AHA and other professionals concerned with heart care will closely scrutinize the long-term benefits of angioplasty performed after three hours after the onset of symptoms to see if there are, indeed, any benefits at all.

The majority of Americans live in areas where the hospital nearest them does not have a cath lab and does not conduct angioplasty programs. The widespread preference of cardiologists to treat heart attack patients in the cath lab has led to their often vigorous promotion of transporting all heart attack patients initially received at hospitals without cath labs to those with labs. The formal version of this movement is to establish what are known as "regional heart centers." The informal version exists in many areas, including Southwest Missouri, where a planned regional program to introduce thrombolysis at community hospitals was abruptly changed by the cardiologists at the base hospital to a program advocating the transportation of all heart attack patients to their hospital for angioplasty.

The major proponents of this transfer system recommend that thrombolysis not be given before departure for the cath lab hospital. You need to know that if this plan is recommended to you, there will be additional time delays before treatment. Besides the door-to-balloon time already described, you would have to add another time interval of fifteen to thirty minutes at the receiving hospital in order to make a decision to transfer you; added to this will be the time to transport you ten, twenty-five, fifty, or even one hundred miles to the cath lab hospital. This may well bring the total symptom-onset-to-balloon time to six hours or more. This is a very long time to wait to get your heart attack treated!

Dr. Richard Conti, editor of the American College of Cardiology's ACCEL Audiotape/CD Service, which reports on current developments in cardiology, is highly critical of this approach. In responding to a report advocating transportation of all patients to cath lab centers without thrombolysis before departure, Conti commented, "Not every place in the United States has facilities where angioplasty can be done. It seems sort of ridiculous to me to transport [heart attack patients] for an hour and then get them into the cath lab. The important thing here is to get the vessel open, and if you can get it open by thrombolysis at [the receiving] hospital, that should be done before sending them on to our cath lab."[23]

In your own decision-making process, it is important that you resist being unduly influenced by the heavily promoted message of "angioplasty for all." Facts provided by the National Registry of Myocardial Infarction, a data-gathering association of 1,600 of the nation's 4,942 hospitals, showed that in a period ending in 1998, only 10 percent of heart attack patients received angioplasty compared with 60 percent who received thrombolysis.[24] This means that by 1998, despite the heavy promotion of angioplasty—despite its proponents referring to it as "the gold standard" in heart attack treatment, a phrase you will still see today—it had not gained universal acceptance in practice. Indeed, in the majority of the cases, it was not used. This reflects the strong disagreement of many in the field with the regional-heart-center concept of angioplasty for all heart attack patients. My own opinion is that transportation of patients to a distant regional center with a cath lab results in care inferior to immediate thrombolysis at the receiving hospital.

There is another drawback to the regional-heart-center concept that concerns me and many others experienced in emergency medicine. Removing heart attack care from hospitals without cath labs would markedly reduce the ability of community hospitals to retain qualified doctors and survive economically. Since this would deprive a great many Americans of the emergency care available at their community hospitals, it would be a great tragedy. The consequences of this are currently being debated in the medical community. Despite the financial incentives of doing "angioplasty for all" (since angioplasty is a far more lucrative procedure for hospitals and doctors than is thrombolysis), I believe that a sufficient number of doctors will recognize the deficiencies of the regional-heart-center model and halt its establishment on a wide scale.

A productive modification of the regional-heart-center plan has come about in Southwest Missouri. It is instructive about how you might choose your treatment in the event that you experience the early warning signs of a heart attack and go to a nearby community hospital that does not have a cath lab. In urban Springfield and the large suburban and rural area surrounding it, there are eighteen hospitals. Of the four hospitals in Springfield, two operate large-volume angioplasty services. Three smaller outlying hospitals perform angioplasties, one only during daytime hours, with thrombolysis for night arrivals. In writing this book, I interviewed members of the staff at all of these hospitals.

Of the thirteen without cath labs, one hospital treats heart attack patients with thrombolysis and continues full treatment there, later referring selected patients to cath lab hospitals for consultation. Eleven of the remaining twelve hospitals give all acute heart attack patients thrombolysis on arrival, and then refer them to cath lab hospitals. The twelfth refers all acute heart attack patients to a cath lab hospital but does not give them thrombolysis before departure. All patients from hospitals more than thirty miles from a cath lab hospital are transported there by helicopter.

Dr. Ron Smalling, a cardiologist at St. John's in Springfield, a major cath lab hospital, reports that St. John's does not do angiograms on arrival of patients who have had thrombolysis at other hospitals because of the increased bleeding that occurs if resulting angioplasty is done so soon after thrombolysis. He reports that angiography on these patients is performed one or more days after arrival. He estimates that in 60 percent of the cases, angiograms reveal that the artery has been reopened by thrombolysis. Data were not available from community hospitals to show whether those whose arteries had not been reopened had arrived at the hospitals at a suitably early time, an important missing piece of information because of the lower rate of success with later treatment.[25]

Interestingly, thrombolysis is used far less frequently for emergency heart attack patients who come directly to the St. John's emergency room. Dr. Scott McMurray reports that for these patients, thrombolysis is given "about once every other year."[26]

I would like to make several important observations about what I learned, and what you can learn, from this informal study. First, thrombolysis can be administered by community hospital physicians soon after patient arrival. Second, Smalling estimates that thrombolysis opens arteries in 60 percent of the cases, and he is a very active member of the interventional cardiology staff at a major hospital. Therefore, his estimate that thrombolysis achieves successful results in a majority of cases is a testament to the value of initial and immediate thrombolysis at the community hospital. Third, it is highly significant that the staff at St. John's considers it acceptable to delay angiography for patients receiving thrombolysis one or more days after arrival. This raises the extremely important possibility of delaying transfer of patients until the day following the heart attack or even a day or two later for daytime transportation by ground ambulance. This would be much less stressful than travel by helicopter, especially helicopter transportation at night. Also, patients appreciate having their personal physician involved with more of their care, which can be accomplished at community hospitals. The cost saving of avoiding helicopter charges is another factor. Finally, it is vital to note that if thrombolysis is successful in opening the artery, there is a cost saving to the patient, not to mention the personal satisfaction of the patient in avoiding angioplasty, an invasive procedure. This finding brings us back to the early years of thrombolysis, when angiography after thrombolysis was carried out only if symptoms persisted or were induced by stress testing. In my opinion, this practice deserves reconsideration.

What Is the Best Treatment If You Have a Heart Attack?

Now that you have learned about the current state of thinking about coronary balloon angioplasty and thrombolysis as treatments for a heart attack, here is a summary of what your priorities must be if you need emergency heart care. First, your goal must be to get treatment within the golden hour, the first sixty minutes of your symptoms. I am convinced that a great many of you can accomplish this. It requires that, on experiencing early warning signs, you immediately chew an adult-size uncoated aspirin and with a call to your doctor or on your own initiative get to the nearest community hospital by the quickest and most appropriate means available for immediate thrombolysis. Remember that the benefits of thrombolysis are proven to continue, to a decreasing degree, to the end of the third hour of symptoms. Second, refuse to agree to be transported to another hospital without thrombolysis if you are eligible for it (as mentioned, a small number of you will not be good candidates). Third, remember that the local hospital staff (and your personal physician, if your health care plan permits) can manage your daily care through discharge unless consultation is needed sooner, and a decision about transfer for angiography can be made at the time of discharge. Last, if your nearest hospital is a large facility with a cath lab and you arrive within the golden hour, the second hour, or the third hour of symptoms, it is very likely that it will be proposed to take you to the cath lab without thrombolysis. Even if you arrive at the hospital within the first sixty minutes of symptoms, adding the usual door-to-balloon time in the reported 70 percent of cath lab hospitals places you in the lab very near, at, or beyond the three-hour point, which Gersh says "is too late to make a difference." You will also recall Weaver's statements about the impossibility of getting into the cath lab early. You have every right to request, and to receive, thrombolysis if it is suitable.

If thrombolysis is given and an ECG shows that the artery has not been opened (an unlikely outcome if thrombolysis is given early), a decision may be made to take you to the cath lab for "rescue" angioplasty. The value of this approach is debatable, and reports of trial studies of this practice are conflicting. Since a substantial number of people are confronted with the need to accept or reject this treatment, I am going to explain it in some detail.

The first problem may be slowness of the emergency room physician to recognize failure of the ECG abnormalities to decrease. (If angioplasty is to be done as a "rescue," it must be done as promptly as possible.) Next, since the majority of patients receiving thrombolysis are treated in hospitals without cath labs, a rescue angioplasty decision often necessitates transfer to a cath lab hospital that may not be ideally prepared to urgently carry out this procedure. I have already discussed the increased risk of bleeding during angioplasty soon after thrombolysis treatment, which introduces further delay. I have not seen a report definitively stating how long is required for this increased bleeding risk to subside. The rescue process, whether carried out in the hospital that directly received the patient or in a referral hospital, extends the symptom-onset-to-balloon time far beyond the three-hour point after which there is usually little muscle remaining to salvage. There is also some unavoidable risk from the angioplasty procedure itself.

To help clarify this important and complex issue, researchers D. R. Holmes Jr. and B. J. Gersh of the Mayo Clinic and S. G. Ellis of the Cleveland Clinic reported a review of older and recent rescue trials in April 2006.[27] None of the three recent trials showed that rescue angioplasty reduced deaths. The doctors recommended that the procedure be undertaken *only* in those patients who continue to have symptoms after the thrombolysis treatment (indicating the possibility that some living muscle remains that might be saved by reopening the partially or completely blocked artery by balloon). They conclude that for rescue angioplasty to be effectively implemented, the medical community has to institute clear guidelines for selecting patients, for staff training, for moving patients, and for assessing outcomes, and emergency room physicians need to be vigilant about whether thrombolysis has been effective with a given patient so that immediate action may be taken if it has not succeeded.

You need to have this information ahead of time so that if you are in a situation in which rescue angioplasty is recommended to you, you can make a more informed decision about accepting or rejecting it. The fact that rescue angioplasty may be problematic should not deter you from accepting thrombolysis; remember that receiving it early is far more successful in the lifesaving and disability-reducing preservation of heart muscle than with the standard angioplasty after three hours.

If you arrive at your community hospital after the first three hours of symptoms, thrombolysis may still be of some benefit and should be given. Some advocate treatment as late as after six hours of symptoms. A decision about transfer to a cardiac hospital for angiograms can be made after full treatment unless earlier consultation is needed.

Patients arriving at the local hospital at any time in obviously serious condition should be transported at once to a major medical center hospital because special procedures available only at these tertiary hospitals (such as treatment of blood pressure emergencies) may be lifesaving. Whether you should have thrombolysis before transfer is a decision the emergency room doctor will help you make.

If you arrive at a cath lab hospital after three hours of symptoms, the benefits from either type of treatment are very limited and not greatly different, as Gersh points out. Remember, research shows that angioplasty at this point will very likely not reduce your chance of dying in the acute attack.[28] It seems to me that the short- and long-term benefits that some attribute to doing angioplasty at this point could be accomplished more conveniently and effectively—and with far less stress to the patient—by giving thrombolysis and later following that electively with angiograms to determine if there is residual artery narrowing that some believe should be dilated by angioplasty with the possibility of reducing future risk. As mentioned, the actual effectiveness of angioplasty to reduce future risk remains to be proven and is still being debated. Above all, keep in mind the most important fact: weighing the evidence, research findings indicate it is not which treatment you choose, *but how soon you receive it!*

In the next chapter, I will discuss another alternative in acute heart attack treatment: the infrequent need for heart surgery.

Chapter 10

Coronary Artery Surgery

There is no more fitting way to introduce you to the fantastic world of coronary artery surgery, the most common type of which is bypass surgery, than to quote the *Texas Heart Institute Journal*'s tribute to Dr. Rene G. Favaloro, who was responsible for so much of it:

> Rene G. Favaloro moved to the Cleveland Clinic in 1962 and with him came a wind of change that was to reshape cardiac surgery forever. With his cherished colleagues, Effler, Sones, Proudfit, Groves, Sheldon, and countless others, he contributed to the double internal mammary artery-myocardial implantation by the Vineberg method, and, subsequently, in May 1967, he reconstructed the right coronary artery by saphenous vein graft interposition. These milestones set the stage for aortocoronary saphenous vein bypass grafting in October 1967. Several other breakthroughs rapidly followed: the application of the bypass technique to the left coronary artery, the combination of coronary artery bypass grafting with left ventricular reconstruction and valve repair or replacement, and finally, by December 1967, a double bypass to the right coronary artery and the anterior descending branch of the left coronary artery. Emergency coronary artery bypass grafting in patients with acute myocardial infarction soon became Favaloro's next focus. In 1970, he was influenced by the work of George Green in New York City and began using the direct mammary-coronary anastomosis with a few modifications, which popularized it. In June 1971 Favaloro decided to leave the Cleve-

> land Clinic and return to Argentina, where he created a medical center, a teaching unit, a research department, and, finally, an Institute of Cardiology and Cardiovascular Surgery. To all these medical achievements, add integrity, courage, honesty, and humility, and the result is a man who will never be forgotten.[1]

This testimonial to Favaloro was well earned, because his introduction of coronary artery surgery revolutionized heart care. Indeed, today coronary artery surgery is the most frequent operation performed on the heart (fig. 10.1). It is time-tested, is highly successful, and usually prolongs and improves life. It is most often carried out to relieve angina resulting from coronary artery narrowing, but is occasionally needed in managing acute heart attacks.

The most recent figures available indicate that 427,000 people per year have coronary artery bypass operations.[2] With so many in potential need of this operation, you need to know more about it. As you have learned, the chest discomfort known as angina is caused by cholesterol narrowing the matchstick-size artery fuel lines to the heart muscle, and this may lead to heart attacks. Coronary artery surgery creates a detour around the obstruction, using a leg vein or chest-wall artery. Vein grafts are attached to the aorta just above the heart and reach beyond the obstruction. The artery grafts extend from their chest-wall origin to below the blockage. By circumventing the obstruction, both types of grafts remarkably restore blood flow to the heart muscle downstream. Obstructions may involve all three of the heart's arteries and even some branches, and may require as many as six or seven grafts.

A surgeon requires vast experience to perfect the skill of rapidly attaching the grafts with tiny stitches without the occurrence of leakage. Results are usually excellent, relieving angina and permitting increased activity. Most patients leave the hospital within a week, and many formerly disabled patients return to work.

Benefits from the surgery may be more complete and longer lasting than those from balloon angioplasty, but costs are greater. Most of those who undergo the surgery are repaid for its considerable cost by regaining their earning power.

A small percentage of grafts become obstructed (or occluded) during the first year. A more important problem following the operation is the possible progression of atherosclerosis, which narrows arteries

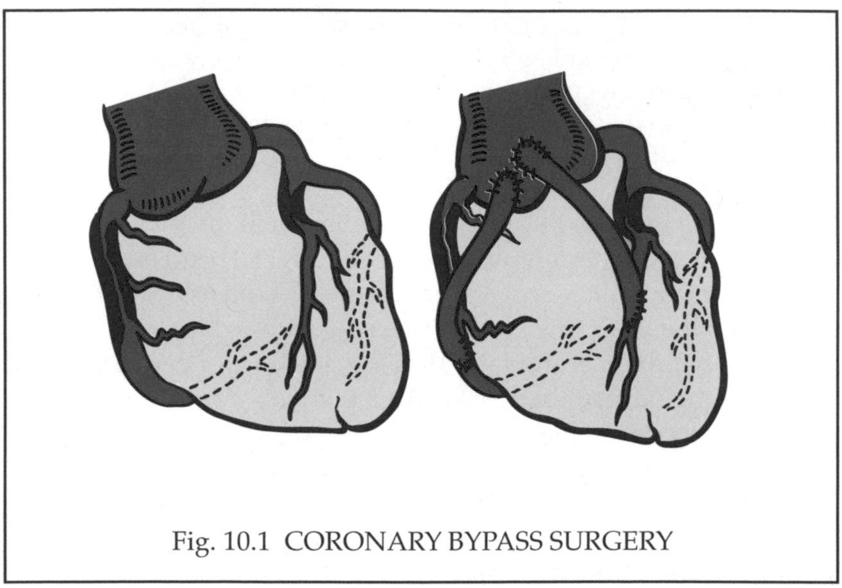

Fig. 10.1 CORONARY BYPASS SURGERY

that were open at the time of surgery and also obstructs the vein or artery grafts. Atherosclerosis of grafts can begin as soon as one year following the surgery and is increasingly frequent after seven to ten years.

The standard time-honored surgical approach to the heart is through a vertical breastbone-splitting incision that gives the surgeon excellent access. The heartbeat is stopped by chemical means, and circulation is maintained by the heart-lung bypass machine, permitting relatively unlimited time for the procedure. Some surgeons operate through the standard sternum-splitting incision but do not stop the heart. With this approach, a device is placed against the surface of the heart to prevent movement at the site of the operation. This is known as "beating-heart surgery." It makes it unnecessary to stop the heart and sustains circulation during the procedure without the heart-lung pump. The continuation of the normal heartbeat eliminates the occasional complications—such as stroke—from the coronary bypass procedure. Another approach is operating through much smaller incisions between the ribs with or without stopping the heart. However, most surgeons continue to use the original traditional method.

After bypass surgery, there are well-known methods for slowing the progression of atherosclerosis that threatens to occlude the grafts and obstruct vessels not narrowed at the time of surgery, but often these methods are not put into practice. It is regrettable that a very significant percentage of bypass operations now being done are performed to reopen obstructed grafts or to bypass new obstructions in other vessels after an initial bypass surgery. Too often, patients believe they have been cured by their first surgery only to recognize later that the problem has recurred. I will discuss today's preventative methods for slowing the progression of atherosclerosis in Part V. Until coronary disease can be eliminated by prevention, early diagnosis and the types of medical and surgical treatments I have described can provide gratifying results.

Part III

The Causes of Heart Attacks and Other Atherosclerotic Diseases

CHAPTER 11

Risk Factors for Heart Attacks and Other Atherosclerotic Diseases

As you know, diseases of the arteries are called atherosclerotic (or arteriosclerotic) diseases. In Part I, I explained the physical nature and structures of the coronary artery narrowings that lead to heart attacks. In this part I am going to look more deeply into the risk factors that influence heart attacks, not only so that you will better understand their causes but, more important, as a foundation for understanding how heart attacks and other atherosclerotic diseases, including many types of strokes, can be prevented.

My initiation into the subject of heart disease came in 1934 when, during my first week in college, at age fifteen, I received a wonderful book, *The Mystery and Magic of Medicine.* As the book made clear, much about heart disease was, indeed, a mystery. Later that year, my biology professor, under whom I was fortunate to serve as a student faculty assistant, died of a heart attack while he was still in his thirties. It was diagnosed by my uncle and benefactor, Dr. E. E. Glenn, who provided my room and board in return for my helping in his office. This help included my operating his newfangled machine, the electrocardiograph. Reading *The Mystery and Magic of Medicine,* losing my college mentor to a heart attack, and doing electrocardiograms for my uncle's patients inspired me to observe and participate in unraveling some of the mysteries of heart attacks.

Since I began my practice in 1947, many of the mysteries have been solved. As a cardiologist it is thrilling to have worked with each new discovery immediately after it was made and to contribute to advances in cardiac patient care. It is particularly thrilling that medical science's increased understanding of the causes of heart attacks has led to lifesaving leaps in understanding the factors that put people at risk for an attack.

The list below shows the generally recognized risk factors for heart attacks, strokes, and other atherosclerotic diseases. Heading the list are the blood lipid abnormalities (cholesterol and triglycerides), cigarette smoking, and hypertension (high blood pressure). Because of their importance, these have long been called the "big three." If you have all three, you have a tenfold greater risk of having a heart attack than if you have none of them. There is now great interest in another abnormality, an excess of the amino acid homocysteine, but at present it does not seem to be a risk factor (see Chapter 14).

- high LDL cholesterol
- low HDL cholesterol
- high triglycerides
- cigarette smoking
- elevated blood pressure
- family history of atherosclerosis or blood lipid abnormality
- male gender in and of itself (even prior to midlife)
- women's postmenopausal state
- diabetes
- excess weight
- physical inactivity
- age—men forty-five or over; women fifty-five or over
- insulin resistance

Recently, the term *metabolic syndrome* has come to be used for a combination of risks and conditions caused by excess weight and physical inactivity, as well as possible genetic factors, which respond positively to weight loss and exercise. These factors appear in slightly different form in the above list, but since metabolic syndrome is becoming an increasingly popular concept, it is important for you to know what it consists of:

- abdominal obesity
- abnormal blood lipids

* elevated triglycerides
* increased small LDL particles
* low HDL cholesterol
* elevated blood pressure
* insulin resistance with or without glucose intolerance (prediabetes or diabetes)

In the following chapters, I will first look at the nature of cholesterol and triglycerides. Because of recent interest in homocysteine excess, I will also discuss it in some detail. The treatment of cholesterol and triglyceride abnormalities—and a full discussion of treating other risk factors, including metabolic syndrome—is presented in Part V, on prevention.

CHAPTER 12

The Cholesterol Problem

Blood fats, also known as lipids or lipoproteins, are of several types, the most well known of which is cholesterol. By now, almost everyone has heard that cholesterol is associated with heart disease. Is cholesterol entirely a villain? No. Cholesterol is a natural substance manufactured in the liver, chiefly from food, and has significant beneficial functions. These include participating in the production of adrenal and sex hormones, nerve-channel sheaths, protective walls for other bodily tissues, and bile acids for digestion and serving as a tissue nutrient throughout the body. The problem is that more than half the U.S. population has too much cholesterol of the wrong kind—which is what makes cholesterol a factor in atherosclerotic diseases.

How do cholesterol abnormalities develop? They develop from a combination of inherited traits and lifestyle choices.

Genetic versus Lifestyle Influences on Cholesterol

With today's increased understanding of traits that are genetically inherited, there is much discussion about the relationship between inherited factors that increase the risk of heart attacks (and other atherosclerotic diseases) and risk factors acquired, or developed, as a result of living habits, especially dietary, and such conditions as weight excess, physical inactivity, and diabetes.

Inherited and acquired factors affect a variety of other risks, particularly cholesterol and other lipid abnormalities. Since inherited and acquired factors greatly influence each other, they must be considered together. For example, a genetic trait can worsen a cholesterol problem caused primarily by an unhealthy lifestyle, such as improper diet and too little physical activity; conversely, whereas healthy personal habits can favorably modify inherited tendencies so that they are less harmful, unhealthy personal habits can cause inherited tendencies to be more harmful.

Although lifestyle changes and medications may offset genetic influences to varying degrees, these influences cannot as yet be entirely eliminated. Thus, treatment and prevention of heart attacks, strokes, and other cardiovascular diseases are inevitably influenced by matters over which we do not have complete control.

The breakthrough good news is that research and clinical trials have now provided us with a far better understanding of abnormalities in the blood fats cholesterol and triglyceride and how to deal with these abnormalities. This means the opportunity to achieve unprecedented success in preventing cardiovascular death and disability. It also means the opportunity to achieve unprecedented success in preventing death and disability from strokes since, as you will learn in Part IV, most strokes are atherosclerotic in nature because they, too, are caused by narrowing of the arteries.

Fundamental to dealing with the cholesterol problem in the United States is recognizing that unlike undeveloped nations and those with certain differences in dietary practices, Americans are habituated to an excessive intake of animal fat, from which we make cholesterol. (Another factor that accompanies excessive intake of animal fat and causes cholesterol abnormalities is the cholesterol already in these animals that we do not need since our bodies can make enough without taking in any cholesterol from outside.)

Along with excessive intake of animal fat, Americans are also habituated to an excessive intake of total calories, which also increases cholesterol production. An additional source of cholesterol problems that can be very serious if left unattended is the genetic inheritance of undesirable patterns of blood-fat production in the liver. These inherited patterns are undesirable because they produce an unhealthy combination of the types of cholesterol: too little of the type of cholesterol we want and too much of the type we do not want.

Cholesterol Types

It is now common knowledge that there are two major types of cholesterol: low-density lipoprotein, or LDL, the "bad" cholesterol (the type we do not want), and high-density lipoprotein, or HDL, the "good" cholesterol (the type we do want). Most people do not realize, however, that each of these cholesterol types has specific ingredients that are important to know about, and that it is also important to know about the other substances involved in atherosclerosis that either stand alone or exist in conjunction with LDL or HDL or both.

Knowing about these basic types of lipoproteins is vital to your health. I will present these lipid substances in summary form so you can make sure that you are tested for them and so that you and your doctor can discuss the results. If your doctor tests for more than these basic types, that is fine, but they are the minimum that you should be tested for. The knowledge you gain about these matters enhances your relationship with your physician. Equally vital is that if you are being treated for an elevated cholesterol level, and in the early weeks you do not respond to treatment as well as expected, you must see if your initial examination tested for all these lipoproteins. If not, further testing should be done. An informed patient is a stimulant to better service. Regrettably, despite the heavy promotion of information about cholesterol, a substantial proportion of U.S. patients visiting their doctor for checkups do not get cholesterol tests or do not get the complete range of tests. Knowing what to ask for will help you get what you need. (As a further aid, see the tabular summary of tests in Appendix A.)

LDL Cholesterol

LDL cholesterol has been given the most attention in the media as a culprit in causing heart attacks. LDL circulates throughout the body as a nutrient to tissues. However, when oxidized (a process of adding oxygen similar to the rusting of metal) it can become attached to the artery wall, creating the deposits known as plaques, discussed in Part I. In time, LDL also accumulates within these plaques as pools of liquid fat covered by thin fibrous caps. These caps are prone to rupture, causing blood to clot at that location in the artery.

Not only does the depositing of LDL continue over the years, but the scar tissue from healing the cracks in the artery lining and the resultant blood clots cause a thickening of the plaques, contributing to the progressive narrowing of the channel. The clotting of blood at these cracks in the artery wall may be sufficient to obstruct blood flow completely, causing a heart attack. The depositing of LDL cholesterol, which may begin in infancy or early childhood as "fatty streaks," is present in the arteries of the majority of individuals by early adulthood.

The degree of increase in the total quantity of LDL over the normal range (see the chart later in this chapter) has long been considered the way to evaluate the risk it poses for creating atherosclerosis. Thus, the more abnormal, or elevated, the level of LDL, the greater risk it poses.

Additionally, it has recently been discovered that there are two different types of LDL: subclass A and subclass B, each exhibiting complex differences in structure and behavior. Subclass B cholesterol particles are smaller and more dense than A particles and are commonly referred to as the "small dense LDL." The reason it is crucial for you to know this is that each of us usually has a predominance of just one type, and there are major differences in the treatment needed for subclass A and the treatment needed for subclass B.

These differences in treatment for A and B patients make it extremely important, if you are found to have an excessive level of LDL, to know your subclass prior to starting treatment. Subclass identification is by the blood test known as "gradient gel electrophoresis," or LDL-GGE. This test has not yet become a routine part of the public screenings that are conducted by hospitals and civic organizations, so you may need to request it from your doctor before treatment is prescribed. If you start treatment (see Part V) and in the early weeks do not respond adequately, you should be tested for all the basic lipoproteins and must also have subclass testing because this may well be the reason you are not responding.

HDL Cholesterol

HDL has emerged as equal in importance to LDL. Reduced levels are a serious atherosclerosis, heart attack, and stroke risk, especially in conjunction with even moderately elevated triglycerides (see Chapter 13). HDL serves as a scavenger, removing LDL particles from the artery walls and returning them to the liver, taking them out of circulation. As the name "high-density lipoprotein" implies, HDL particles are dense, heavier in weight than the larger, less dense, "fluffier" LDL particles.

To a degree, HDL deficiency is genetically influenced, although this inherited tendency may be worsened by acquired problems such as excess weight and physical inactivity. A deficiency in HDL means that more LDL is allowed to remain attached to artery walls. The protection provided by normal or increased levels of HDL is illustrated by the low incidence of heart attacks in premenopausal women, who have higher HDL levels because of the influence of estrogen but lose that protection at menopause, leading to a sharp increase in heart attacks in postmenopausal women (see Chapter 40).

Just as LDL has subclasses A and B, HDL has component fractions known as HDL2 and HDL3. These are measurable by a variety of gradient gel electrophoresis known as the HDL-GGE test. HDL2 is generally believed to be more protective than HDL3, but until that question is resolved by the researchers, you and your doctor should be guided by your HDL total figure. The apoprotein A-1 test is helpful in making that measurement. (I will present figures for total cholesterol, HDL, and LDL later in this chapter.)

VLDL Cholesterol

VLDL, or very low-density lipoprotein, is also known as non-HDL cholesterol. Normally present in the human body in amounts of up to thirty milligrams, excesses of this lipoprotein appear in individuals with very high triglycerides (see next chapter), and these elevations participate in causing atherosclerosis. The total cholesterol is the sum of LDL, HDL, and VLDL values.

Other Significant Lipids

Lipoprotein (a), or LP(a), commonly called "LP little a," leads the list of other lipids that are associated with heart disease and other atherosclerotic diseases, and is present in about one-third of coronary artery disease patients. A genetically transmitted substance, LP(a) consists of a union between certain LDL particles and what is known as apoprotein A or apo A (a component of blood fats).

Some authorities report that LP(a) facilitates blood clotting, accelerates the thickening of atherosclerotic plaques, and increases the oxidation of LDL that is necessary before it can become attached to artery walls. General population studies show that individuals with the higher level of this lipoprotein have a 70 percent greater likelihood of developing coronary artery disease. It is not included in public screenings, but testing is now widely available. Make sure your doctor obtains this test, especially if you have any other risks.

In addition to the apo A described above in relation to uniting with LDL particles to form LP(a), additional apoproteins that may be associated with coronary disease are apoproteins B, C-H, and E2, -3, and -4. Testing for this complex array of substances may require the services of a lipid specialist. The degree to which your physician will choose to assay these agents will probably depend on how well you respond to treatment based on the other set of factors described in this section. The summary of tests in Chapter 37 lists the availability of these special measurements, and Appendix A lists their approximate costs.

Proper Amounts of Cholesterol

Looking at your cholesterol level to see whether it is cause for concern requires what I call "patient mathematics." Until dangerous atherosclerotic complications occur, cholesterol (and triglyceride) excesses are entirely without symptoms. Often, the first knowledge a person may have of a problem is when the heart attack, stroke, or need for coronary bypass surgery occurs because of artery obstruction by a blood clot or by a cholesterol plaque. Elevated lipid levels are all the more important when they occur in conjunction with other risk factors: cigarette smoking, hypertension, excess weight, physical inactivity, diabetes, and family history of heart or other atherosclerotic disease.

After you have learned your cholesterol levels, see where they fit in the following tables. Remember that low-density lipoprotein excess or high-density lipoprotein deficiency places you at risk of a heart attack, stroke, or other atherosclerotic disease.

Total cholesterol values in adults	
Desirable	Less than 200
Borderline high	200–239
High	More than 240

Low-density lipoprotein (LDL) values for men and women	
Optimal	Less than 100
Near or above optimal	100–129
Borderline high	130–59
High	160–89
Very high	More than 190

The National Cholesterol Education Program (NCEP) states that with zero or one risk factor, the desirable LDL level is 160 or below and that with two or more risk factors, the level should be 130 or below. Some advocate lower values than these. All authorities agree that everyone with known atherosclerotic disease should have their LDL reduced to 100 or below, and some advocate considering a level of 70 for such individuals.

High-density lipoprotein (HDL) values	
Normal	
Men	45 or above
Women	55 or above
Low for either	below 40
High for either	above 60

Getting the Right Tests at the Right Times

Since a test is required to discover excess LDL or a deficiency in HDL, and no law demands these examinations, you will have to take action to be tested. If your doctor does not routinely test your blood-fat levels, you should request that he or she does so. Although everyone should have a personal physician, if you do not have one, you should consider other ways of obtaining cholesterol screening (see Chapter 37).

As of 2001, the NCEP guidelines stipulate that a complete assay of cholesterol measurements, including total cholesterol, LDL cholesterol, HDL cholesterol, and triglycerides, should be done for every person by age twenty and repeated every five years. It is my opinion that every person over the age of twenty should ideally have these tests performed annually; if you know you have lipid abnormalities, you must be under a doctor's care and make sure that these tests are performed as frequently as needed.

Because of the early childhood onset of atherosclerosis, and the treatments available for it even for children (see Chapters 34, 36, and 37), most authorities advise that any child with a family history of heart disease, blood lipid abnormality, or other risk factors should have the full assay by age two. A serious problem with this plan is that these factors may be present in a child's family but may not have come to light by the time the child is two years old. Consequently, some authorities say that testing only those with a known family history misses half the children who actually have a positive family history, and they therefore advocate full assay preschool testing of all children. I know that many people will be surprised by the idea of starting blood-fat testing so early in a child's life, but it is vital information because you want to raise your children in the healthiest way possible.

What is involved in blood-fat testing? Until recently, the gold standard of accuracy in measuring cholesterol and other lipids was a test requiring the use of blood drawn by a needle from an arm vein. Although this is still the most common practice, a new method has been devised whereby a small drop of blood obtained by finger-stick can be used to give accurate results with the proper equipment. With this method, the report is provided in printed form in five minutes (see Chapter 37).

Whereas HDL can be measured along with total cholesterol, adding LDL cholesterol and triglycerides to the assay, as now advised by the NCEP, requires that the blood specimen for testing be drawn after at least a twelve-hour fast. (The few additional dollars' cost of the full assay is well worthwhile.) Results should be reported to you in actual numbers with appropriate explanation. Abnormal results should be rechecked at least once.

Remember that if you have a public screening for lipid levels, LDL subclass determinations will not be part of the screening. If you find that you have an LDL elevation, make sure that your doctor orders an LDL subclass assay for you.

CHAPTER 13

The Triglyceride Story

After many years of uncertainty, the blood fat triglyceride has come to be recognized as also contributing to atherosclerotic diseases. Triglycerides are partly derived from carbohydrates (sugar and starch) and serve as a storage form of the fat and carbohydrates we eat. The amount of triglycerides in the bloodstream is increased by excessive weight, particularly from excessive sugar and starch, and by physical inactivity, diabetes, overuse of alcohol, and certain inherited traits.

Triglycerides do not participate in the formation of atherosclerotic plaques (low-density lipoprotein cholesterol deposits), which is why many authorities believed for a time that elevated triglycerides had little connection with atherosclerosis. Much remains to be learned about how triglycerides do their harm. One theory is that as they are being transported through the body as a food source, they serve as a carrier for cholesterol. This theory suggests that an excess of triglycerides could deliver an increased amount of cholesterol to locations where it could attach to the artery wall to form obstructive plaques.

Triglyceride excess can be found only by blood testing of the lipid fractions. It is not revealed by simply a measurement of total cholesterol, the kind of screening program frequently available at public fairs. A twelve-hour fast is required prior to triglyceride testing. Since a separate test is required for triglycerides, the triglyceride level is reported separately from the cholesterol level.

What Is a Healthy Triglyceride Level?

Opinions have differed about what level of triglycerides in the blood constitutes an excess, but in 2001 the NCEP released the following figures arrived at by their panel of experts:

Normal	Up to 150
Borderline high	150–99
High	200–499
Very high	Above 500

One of the most common blood-lipid patterns associated with heart attacks and strokes is the combination of slight to moderate triglyceride elevations with deficiency of the "good" high-density lipoprotein cholesterol. This combination is a risk separate from the risk posed by the total cholesterol levels alone.

Inherited triglyceride excess may take a number of forms—some with cholesterol excess, some without it. One kind can cause severe inflammation of the pancreas, known as pancreatitis, which may lead to diabetes.

It is important to remember that the NCEP now recommends full assay testing, to include triglycerides in addition to total LDL and HDL cholesterols, regardless of whether the examination is in a physician's office, at a public screening, or at a commercial facility.

How are abnormal triglyceride values corrected? Primarily by weight reduction, moderation of sugar and starch intake, and restriction of alcohol usage to a maximum of two ounces per day. Medications may also be needed. I will discuss all of these treatments in Part V, on prevention.

CHAPTER 14

Homocysteine Excess

A New Puzzle

When I listed the risk factors for heart and other atherosclerotic diseases, I told you that there has been a great deal of interest in homocysteine excess, but I did not list it as a risk factor. In this chapter, I will explain why.

Homocysteine is an amino acid (a building block of protein). It is derived from another amino acid, methionine, one of the twenty amino-acid building-block components of human muscle and of other protein in the body. Breakdown of homocysteine as it is used in bodily function yields final products that are eliminated through the kidneys as waste. Homocysteine excess, or hyperhomocysteinemia, results from incomplete breakdown of the homocysteine for excretion, causing a buildup of it in the blood to excessive levels. A special test is required to measure this level.

In the past several years, a flood of medical research established blood homocysteine excess as correlating with atherosclerotic diseases, including heart attacks, strokes, peripheral arterial disease, and kidney failure.[1] Homocysteine excess is also associated with increased blood clotting in veins of the legs, called thrombophlebitis, and in pulmonary embolism, a major death risk that consists of the dislodgement of these clots into the lungs.

In 1997, the American Heart Association declared homocysteine a close second to cholesterol as a risk factor for heart attacks. Other authorities considered homocysteine a risk factor as important as smoking and said it increased the risks caused by smoking and hypertension. When this was the prevailing opinion, the good news seemed to be that homocysteine excess, whether present through genetic abnormalities or dietary deficiency, can be corrected through increasing intake of vitamins B_6, B_{12}, and folic acid. This can be accomplished through a combination of increasing intake of foods rich in these nutrients and taking vitamin supplements. The dietary source of B_{12} is animal protein through the consumption of red meat, poultry, and fish. B_6 is supplied by wheat, vegetables (especially beans), nuts, fruit, cereals, and meat, including chicken, and fish. Folic acid is found in green leafy vegetables, fruit, beans, liver, and yeast.

There is widespread deficiency of B_6 and folic acid because of the marked loss of these vitamins, as well as of B_{12}, in the processing, refining, and preserving of foods in the United States. Even refrigeration causes considerable loss. Thus, to increase these nutrients in your system, in addition to taking vitamin supplements that contain them, your green leafy vegetables should come straight from the garden or be certified organic from an organic market.

It was theorized that if homocysteine excess was lowered by these means, it would also lower heart attack risk. Recent research put this theory to the test—with results that surprised many. The studies showed that although excess homocysteine levels can, indeed, be lowered through increasing intake of B_6, B_{12}, and folic acid, lowered levels do *not* lessen the risk of heart attacks. Thus, it now seems that excess homocysteine, though associated with atherosclerotic diseases, does not *cause* them. Further research will reveal more about this potentially helpful subject.

Part IV

How to Recognize and Respond to the Early Warning Signs of a Stroke or "Brain Attack"

CHAPTER 15

An Urgent Message

Learn the Early Warning Signs of a Stroke

Many people fear having a stroke, but few understand exactly what it is. Even fewer are aware that there are new breakthroughs in stroke treatment and prevention. This part, which encompasses ten chapters, will educate you with this critical information.

Strokes are the third-leading cause of death (following heart attacks and cancer) and the most common cause of disability. The good news is that like heart attacks, strokes have early warning signs that you can learn and heed to prevent death and prevent or minimize disability.

The usual cause of strokes is the obstruction of an artery supplying blood to a portion of the brain, much as blockage of an artery nourishing the heart causes a heart attack. This similarity has led some to refer to a stroke as a "brain attack." A small percentage of strokes result from the rupture of a blood vessel. This is known as a cerebral hemorrhage or a brain hemorrhage. The various causes of strokes or brain attacks will be covered in a crash course in neurology in this and subsequent chapters. This information may be learned—and used—just as you have learned to use the essential information about heart attacks and how to respond to their symptoms.

But before further examining the causes of strokes or discussing treatment and prevention, here is a list of the early warning signs of a stroke. As with heart attacks, knowing these early warning signs

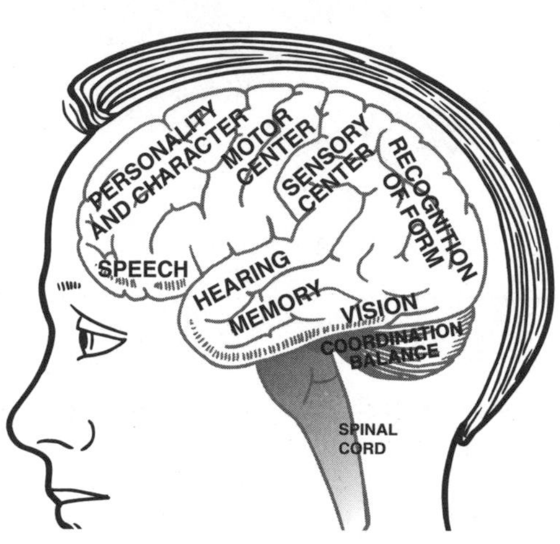

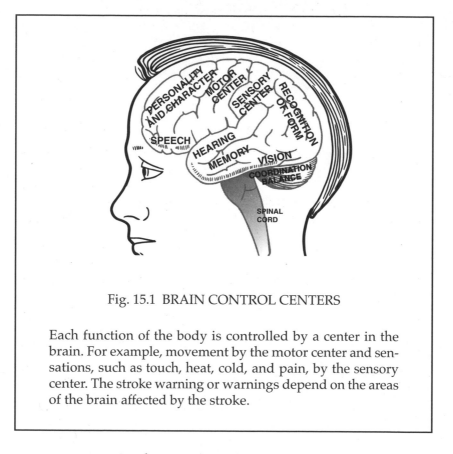

Fig. 15.1 BRAIN CONTROL CENTERS

Each function of the body is controlled by a center in the brain. For example, movement by the motor center and sensations, such as touch, heat, cold, and pain, by the sensory center. The stroke warning or warnings depend on the areas of the brain affected by the stroke.

can save your life. These early warning signs can appear as single symptoms or together:

- sudden weakness or numbness of the face, arm, or leg, usually on one side
- sudden change in eyesight, usually in one eye
- loss of speech or trouble talking or understanding speech
- sudden severe headache with no known cause
- unexplained dizziness, unsteadiness, or falls, especially along with any other symptoms of a stroke

Which of these symptoms is experienced during a stroke is determined by which area of the brain is deprived of blood flow. Figure 15.1 shows the brain control centers that may be affected.

Surveys have shown that 30 percent of Americans do not know even one of these warnings.[1] Taking advantage of the wonderful new treatments and preventive measures requires memorizing and promptly paying attention to these signs.

One reassurance: dizziness alone, without other warning signs, is frequently caused by the troublesome but usually not serious condition known as "inner-ear trouble." A common rule of thumb among physicians is to regard dizziness occurring alone as probably not due to a stroke, but to regard dizziness plus other warnings as possibly indicative of a stroke. Even though this is the case, if dizziness occurs alone or in conjunction with other symptoms, or if any one of the other symptoms occurs, if possible call your doctor. If he or she is not immediately available, or if your health care plan does not permit such an emergency call, get to your hospital emergency room by the quickest means possible.

CHAPTER 16

How to Respond to the Early Warning Signs of a Stroke

On experiencing the early warning signs of a heart attack, you have to go to the nearest hospital as quickly as possible. On experiencing what appear to be the early warning signs of a stroke, *you need to know where you should go for hospital services.* The reason: not all hospitals have the equipment that may be necessary for your care.

The lifesaving and disability-reducing treatment for most acute strokes is the "clot-buster" thrombolysis that is also so effective with heart attacks. With the most common kinds of stroke—those caused by artery obstruction—the blood clot causing the obstruction ideally should be dissolved by drugs within three hours of symptom onset in order to prevent irreversible brain damage. Because thrombolytic agents worsen bleeding if bleeding is already occurring from blood vessel rupture, thrombolysis *must not* be given without a CT or MRI brain scan to rule out bleeding from blood vessel rupture as the cause of the stroke. A CT or MRI brain scan will also identify possible bleeding from recent bodily injury or surgery. Brain-scan equipment is costly and thus not purchased by all hospitals. If your doctor is available to you during a stroke emergency, he or she will know where brain-scan equipment is immediately available. Whether or not your health plan allows your personal physician to attend you in an emergency, *you should find out now which hospitals in your area provide brain-scan services twenty-four hours a day.* Losing time through transfer from one hospital to another when you could have gone directly to

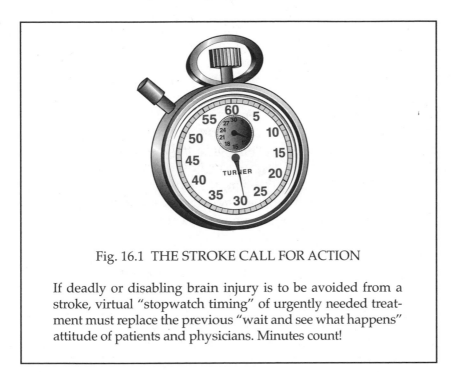

Fig. 16.1 THE STROKE CALL FOR ACTION

If deadly or disabling brain injury is to be avoided from a stroke, virtual "stopwatch timing" of urgently needed treatment must replace the previous "wait and see what happens" attitude of patients and physicians. Minutes count!

the more suitable one might mean needless loss of brain function. Even if your personal physician will not be able to be present in an emergency, you can still get his or her input during an office visit, and, if necessary, you can call hospitals on your own to find out which of them provide brain scans twenty-four hours a day.

Another crucial point: If you are covered by a managed care contract, *obtain an absolute guarantee now that if you have a stroke, you can have immediate access to proper care,* including a CT or MRI brain scan. In the event that your managed care provider will not make this guarantee, then you must ascertain how to obtain and pay for this service on your own initiative. Frequently, hospitals want to be paid in advance when services are not covered by an insurance plan. Fortunately, most hospitals accept payment by credit card. All of this is vital to know in advance. Ideally, as with a heart attack, a patient should arrive at the hospital and receive care for a stroke during the first sixty minutes of symptoms, the golden hour.

Choice of transportation during a suspected stroke follows the same principle as during a possible heart attack: if your doctor is not *immediately* available to advise you, use the quickest means of travel possible to get to the hospital. In rural areas, the family automobile may be fastest, unless in the best judgment of yourself or your family, your condition would prohibit its use. If you go by car during a possible stroke, rest in a semireclining or lying position (in contrast to travel by car during a possible heart attack, when it is best to sit upright). When you have your next appointment, discuss with your doctor what his or her views are about the best form of transportation for you to take to the appropriate hospital if you were to experience what you believe are the symptoms of a stroke.

If you use an ambulance, it is important to know that irrespective of the patient's wishes, some ambulance services are restricted regarding hospitals to which they can transport patients. If you can call your personal physician at the onset of symptoms, he or she can probably eliminate this problem by calling the ambulance and giving orders concerning destination. If a personal physician will not be available to you in an emergency, investigate your local ambulance services now to find out how you can go by ambulance to your hospital of choice should an ambulance be necessary.

In summary, to respond to the early warning signs of a possible stroke, you need (1) a personal physician, if possible, and knowledge about how to make contact with him or her in emergencies, day or night, and (2) knowledge about which hospitals provide the necessary CT brain-scan equipment twenty-four hours per day. If you need an ambulance, you also need to know which hospital the ambulance will take you to in order to make sure you go to a hospital with the proper equipment.

CHAPTER 17

With Stroke Warnings, What Will Happen at the Hospital?

As with heart attacks, emergency room staffs have been trained to operate with stopwatch timing in the event a patient comes in with a suspected stroke. If you have contacted your personal physician, he or she will alert the emergency room to expect your arrival; if you arrive via ambulance, the emergency room will be alerted by the attendants. If you come in on your own, tell the registering nurse that you suspect you are having a stroke and decline to be delayed by registration paperwork. A rapid medical history, requiring no more than five minutes, and an equally rapid neurological and heart examination will be done immediately. These tests will indicate to the emergency room staff whether you have even a small possibility of a stroke.

If it is possible that you are having a stroke, a CT or MRI brain scan must be done *immediately,* day or night. If you arrive at a hospital where this service is not available, ask for immediate transfer to a facility where it is. Do not hesitate to request this.

During this period, your blood will be drawn for tests and an intravenous line will usually be established in anticipation of possible thrombolysis. An electrocardiogram, or heart tracing, will also be taken promptly because of the frequent association of heart disease with strokes. If the findings indicate a stroke and the brain scan shows it not to have been the result of a brain hemorrhage from a ruptured blood vessel, thrombolysis treatment can begin (fig. 17.1).

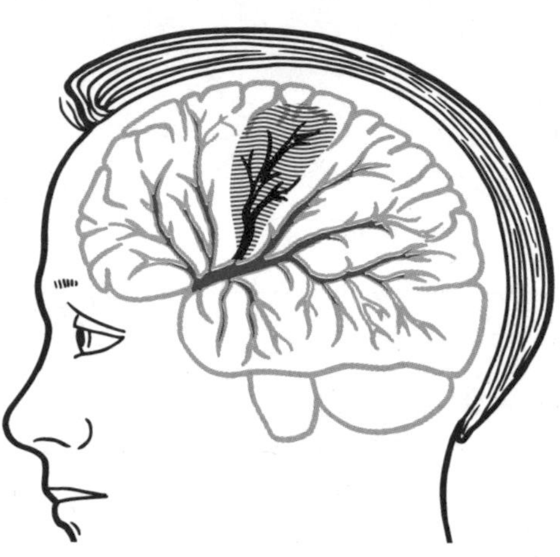

Fig. 17.1 MIDDLE-BRAIN STROKE

The most common stroke location due to brain-artery obstruction by blood clot is the middle brain, which controls motor and sensory centers. Clots here cause weakness or numbness of the opposite side of the body or both. Before "clot-buster" thrombolysis treatment may be used, a CT scan must rule out a hemorrhage.

Research is currently being conducted to determine the best way to administer thrombolysis, which patients are most suitable for treatment with it, and how long after onset of symptoms treatment is beneficial. Research indicates that MRI studies, which can be completed in twenty minutes, may be more accurate than CT scanning to identify the obstructed artery, permitting a direct approach by an arterial catheter. By suction through the catheter, it may be possible to remove the obstructing clot. Injecting the thrombolytic agent through a catheter directly to the clot dissolves it more quickly. Some of these studies show that thrombolysis treatment of strokes affecting the underside of the brain may be beneficial well after three hours of symptom onset.

These continuing advances make it mandatory that you remain informed about which hospitals in your area are best equipped and staffed to care for you in the event of a stroke, even though you may have to travel farther to get there. Your doctor, your local heart association, and your medical society are your best sources of information.

Few procedures in medicine are more gratifying than seeing the dissolving of a clot and the reopening of an artery to the brain or to the heart. That thrombolysis can accomplish this in so many cases may well make it the biggest medical advance of the past century!

For patients who are not eligible for thrombolysis, prompt attention to the stroke can usually make a great difference in the ultimate outcome. Even without thrombolysis, much can be done for brain impairment from stroke. Even if a patient arrives at a hospital later than the three-hour window, treatment is vital. In all patients, correcting of blood pressure abnormality, maintenance of proper breathing, and attention to possible heart rhythm disturbances is carried out.

From the point of your crucial initial treatment forward, management of your care will be up to the judgment of your physician and consultants, possibly including rehabilitation therapists, who may be brought in.

Do not let the results of treatment, regardless of how successful, deter you from taking advantage of the breakthroughs that prevent recurrence of a stroke. I will discuss the types of blood vessel obstructions causing strokes in forthcoming chapters where I will also discuss preventive measures. It is particularly important for you to avoid a first stroke or brain attack by learning and paying attention to the stroke risk factors.

CHAPTER 18

The Primary Stroke Culprit—Atherosclerosis—and Other Causes of Strokes

The chief villain in a stroke or brain attack, accounting for the majority of cases, is atherosclerosis. Fortunately, atherosclerosis is treatable and increasingly preventable. An additional 20 percent of strokes are caused by emboli, blood clots dislodged from the heart either when the heart rhythm disturbance known as atrial fibrillation occurs or after a heart attack. Fifteen percent of strokes result from the rupture of a blood vessel, an event contributed to by congenital abnormality and high blood pressure, causing a hemorrhage (see Chapter 20).

Cholesterol deposits in the artery wall can affect any or all of the vessels in the arterial system nourishing the brain, from the largest to the smallest. The carotid and basilar arteries, carrying blood from the aorta, just above the heart, through the neck into the cranial cavity and on to the branching vessels on and within the brain, are especially vulnerable. In a stroke, the carotid arteries, which cause the pulse in your neck, are most affected. Narrowing of the carotid arteries by atherosclerosis can be readily diagnosed and treated, thus preventing many strokes (see Chapter 22 and Part V on prevention).

Besides the immediate lifesaving and disability-preventing importance of thrombolysis as a treatment for most strokes that are acutely under way, other breakthroughs have led to unprecedented possibilities for stroke prevention. Statin drugs (described in Chapter 35) not only reduce cholesterol and help stop cholesterol deposits from forming but also help prevent the artery lining from making blood clot obstructions and have been shown to reduce strokes by 50 percent. Benefits appear within months of starting the drug treatment.

The lack of public knowledge about strokes—the warning signs, causes, treatment, and prevention—keeps many people from benefiting from some of the most important medical advances of our time. To develop an adequate prevention plan, you must do the following: First, locate a personal physician who is committed to stroke prevention. He or she does not need to be a neurologist. Obtain adequate physical and laboratory examinations, including cholesterol analysis, for discovery of stroke risks. Second, receive long-term *permanent follow-up* by your physician at sufficiently frequent intervals to ensure attention to potential problems. Third, obtain the medications you need. Although expensive, they reduce the long-term costs of care. (Some managed care companies restrict use of such medications, forcing some patients to change care plans and physicians.) Last, continue your medications year-round, if so prescribed. Many patients discontinue their medicine without proper cause within the first twelve months.

CHAPTER 19

Atrial Fibrillation

A Neglected Cause of Strokes

Atrial fibrillation is an irregularity of the heart rhythm that leads to formation of blood clots within the heart. These clots break loose and lodge in arteries throughout the body. Clots pumped into brain arteries cause more than one hundred thousand strokes per year.[1] Half of these strokes could be prevented by an anticoagulant blood-clot-reducing treatment, but currently only half of the patients who need the treatment receive it, and for half of those, the drug dose is inadequate. Awareness of the treatment and the necessity of an adequate dose will stop this from happening to you.

To understand what happens when atrial fibrillation causes a brain attack, let's first review what occurs when the heart is functioning normally. Normally, the heartbeat consists of blood being received by the upper chambers, the right and left atria. The right receives used blood from throughout the body, whereas the left receives refreshed blood after it passes through the lungs. With each beat, the atria pump blood into the lower chambers, the ventricles. The right ventricle pumps used blood through the lungs, and the left pumps the rejuvenated blood throughout the body. When functioning properly, the upper heart chambers empty completely and with no slowing of blood flow, thereby preventing clotting. As you learned in Chapter 1, electrical control by the sinoatrial node regulates the heartbeat. In

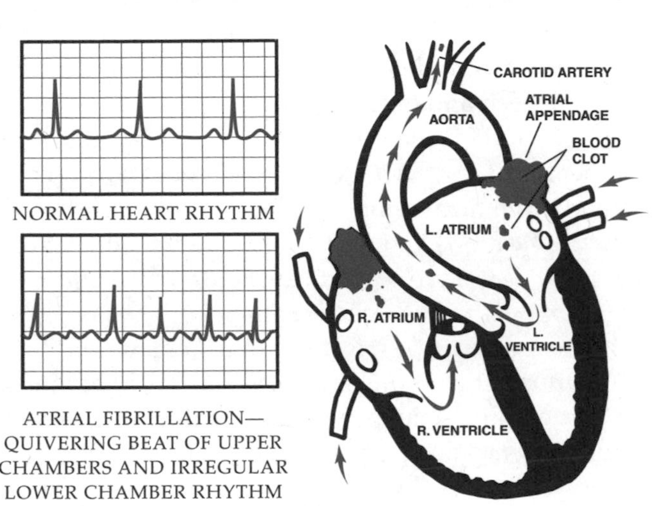

Fig. 19.1 ATRIAL FIBRILLATION AND STROKE

Atrial fibrillation is a change from the regular beating of the upper heart chambers (atria) to an irregular quivering, which incompletely empties them, causing clots around the atrial walls. Clot fragments frequently break loose and are pumped out over the body, often into the brain arteries—a notorious cause of strokes unless treatment is given.

atrial fibrillation, the atria lose electrical control. The quivering motion of the atria that results prevents them from completely emptying with each heartbeat. The blood that remains in the atria clots readily, especially around the atrial walls in protuberances called appendages, where clots loosely adhere (fig. 19.1).

These clots readily break apart, and pieces enter the ventricles. Pieces in the right ventricle are pumped into the lungs, causing blood clots, or a pulmonary embolism. Large pieces of these clots pumped by the left ventricle can obstruct sizable arteries, such as those to the legs. Smaller fragments can enter more narrow vessels, particularly the carotid arteries, which carry blood to the brain. Tiny fragments can pass through to small branches and cause small strokes. Medium fragments can obstruct the carotids near their origin, with devastating results—death or complete paralysis of one side of the body plus possible loss of speech and other effects.

In the event of atrial fibrillation, the first goal is trying to eliminate the irregular beating. On arrival in the emergency room, after testing has determined atrial fibrillation, regulation of the heartbeat will be attempted by medications and electrical cardioversion (utilizing the same machine that is used to correct ventricular fibrillation, the most common cause of death in acute heart attacks).

Restoring a regular heartbeat is difficult to achieve and to sustain. In cases where normal rhythm cannot be started or maintained by medication and cardioversion, increasingly doctors are using surgery or radio frequency ablation, a technique for interrupting nerve pathways involved in the fibrillation.

For those whose atrial fibrillation cannot be corrected or who have recurrence after conversion, reducing the blood's ability to clot is essential. Until recently, aspirin was favored to accomplish this because it is so simple to use. However, studies have proven that the anticoagulant warfarin, marketed as Coumadin, is superior and should be used except in very low-risk patients. Some physicians say that anyone with atrial fibrillation should be on warfarin for life. Although some patients become aware of the irregular beat of atrial fibrillation because they feel it, many do not. This possibility is one of the reasons everyone needs a personal physician and needs to be checked regularly (at *least* annually) rather than first learning of the problem when a stroke occurs or a leg artery becomes blocked.

Outpatient anticoagulant treatment has been available since about 1950, but use is hampered by the amount of attention required from the physician. Risks of bleeding from anticoagulation have caused some physicians to avoid the treatment or not to give a large-enough dose. However, in my extensive observation, the actual instances of occurrence of bleeding from anticoagulation are far less than the number of strokes prevented by it. In some areas, anticoagulant clinics are being set up for treatment. Blood tests at regular intervals are required. If you suspect your heartbeat is "out of tune," see your doctor!

CHAPTER 20

Brain Hemorrhage Strokes

A sudden, often instantaneous, headache at any location—front, back, top, or side of the head—is the most frequent warning sign of a stroke caused by blood vessel rupture. This is commonly called a cerebral hemorrhage or a brain hemorrhage. Any or all of the other stroke warnings I have enumerated may also occur. *Any instant headache, especially if severe, must be considered the result of a cerebral hemorrhage until proven otherwise.*

In half the cases, a vessel on the brain surface has ruptured, which causes bleeding that surrounds and compresses that portion of the brain. This is known as a subarachnoid hemorrhage. In the other half of strokes caused by blood vessel ruptures, bleeding is into the interior of the brain, often very destructive of brain tissue (fig. 20.1). In either type of blood vessel rupture, the most common cause of a stroke is the bursting of an aneurysm, a berrylike bulge of an artery present at birth or developing later. High blood pressure increases the risk of developing aneurysms and makes the rupture of any type of artery-wall weakness more likely. Aneurysms can occur at virtually any location within the head, with the rupture-producing effects dependent on the brain center(s) involved. If diagnosed in time, the majority of aneurysms can be reached surgically and closed.

A less common type of congenital abnormality, arteriovenous malformation (an intermingling of small arteries and veins), can also cause bleeding anywhere within the brain. Prompt examination can

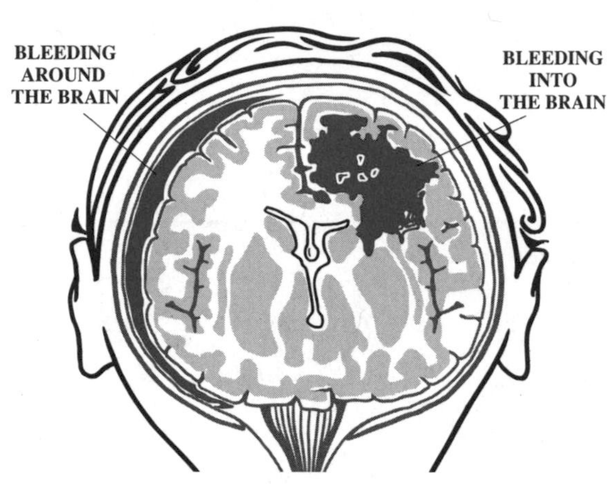

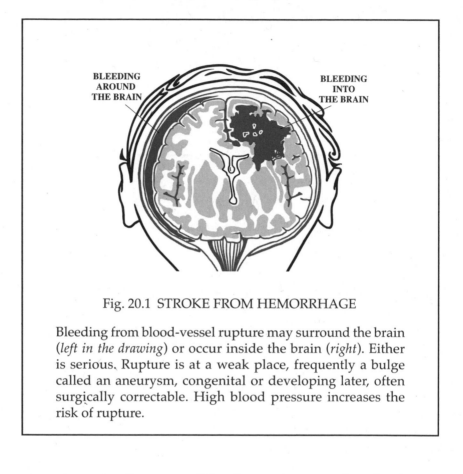

Fig. 20.1 STROKE FROM HEMORRHAGE

Bleeding from blood-vessel rupture may surround the brain (*left in the drawing*) or occur inside the brain (*right*). Either is serious. Rupture is at a weak place, frequently a bulge called an aneurysm, congenital or developing later, often surgically correctable. High blood pressure increases the risk of rupture.

often determine the source of bleeding in time to get beneficial treatment under way.

As mentioned in Chapter 7, there is also a slight chance that thrombolysis treatment for a heart attack (or stroke, see Chapter 17) may cause bleeding that can then cause a brain hemorrhage.

First, a CT brain scan, which usually will disclose bleeding at any location, is done. Another special examination, known as magnetic resonance imaging, may also be used. Angiograms, using dye injections to disclose the presence and location of an aneurysm or an arteriovenous malformation, are necessary in helping to decide whether surgical treatment is possible. Medical management includes correction of high blood pressure (see Chapter 39).

The role of prevention of hemorrhagic stroke has become more and more promising. Today, control of high blood pressure is possible in practically all cases—but it is accomplished in no more than 25 or 30 percent of those needing it. As with control of cholesterol excess, another major stroke prevention measure, if you have high blood pressure, take the necessary steps to control it and prevent a stroke.

CHAPTER 21

TIAs and Stroke Prevention

A transient ischemic attack (TIA) is an important type of early warning sign of a stroke. Indeed, experiencing a TIA is a valuable alert that signals the need to take advantage of measures that are generally highly effective for the prevention of a future stroke. For that reason, I am going to discuss TIAs in some detail.

Ischemic means shortage of blood. TIAs are a shortage of blood to the brain. (This is in contrast with brain injury by hemorrhage from tissue destruction or compression.) When interruption of flow persists three hours or more, brain tissue dies; when the interference with blood flow is temporary and brief, TIAs occur.

TIAs most often result from severe narrowings of the carotid arteries in the neck or higher up in the brain arteries. These narrowings can cause inadequate blood flow to the brain, particularly when the blood pressure drops during sleep or at times of increased need, such as during exercise or excitement. In addition, fragments of cholesterol deposits in the carotids, perhaps with small blood-clot particles, may dislodge and be pumped into the smaller brain-artery branches, producing small strokes or possibly temporary ischemia, a variety of TIA.

With TIAs, exactly the same stroke warnings may occur as those presented for an actual stroke, the difference being duration. Whereas strokes generally cause long-lasting symptoms, symptoms from most TIAs are for five minutes or less, with no symptom lasting more than twenty-four hours.

If even one, and certainly two or more, TIA occurs, your risk of a major stroke in one to two years is high. Of patients having actual or "completed" strokes, approximately 75 percent have had TIAs in the recent past. Some strokes occur soon after TIAs, even during the following weeks or months. Given this, if you experience a TIA, you usually have some time to take corrective action.

The first step is an urgent call to your doctor to obtain an examination as soon as possible. At the examination, your doctor uses a stethoscope to see if he hears a bruit (a sound signaling partial blockage of blood flow) at the side of the neck where the pulse is felt. The loudness of the bruit indicates the severity of the blockage. (This is why as part of your annual or semiannual exam your doctor uses a stethoscope and listens at the side of your neck.) If the stethoscope on the surface of your neck reveals a bruit, your doctor will follow up with other examinations. As described in the next chapter, ultrasound examination of the carotids is usually next. It has become very frequent practice for hospitals and mobile commercial units to conduct screenings including carotid and abdominal-artery ultrasound and a variety of leg-artery examinations. I strongly favor this relatively inexpensive practice.

My primary purpose in focusing on TIAs is to draw your attention to this very rewarding opportunity for action to prevent a fatal or disabling stroke. Committing the early warning signs of stroke to memory is as important as learning the early warning signs of a heart attack—and may well save your life, save the life of a loved one, or prevent paralysis and other severe effects of a stroke.

CHAPTER 22

Neck-Artery Surgery

Another Milestone

Analysis of thousands of cases has proven the enormous benefit of surgically removing cholesterol narrowings of the carotid arteries in the neck. This surgery particularly benefits patients with severe obstructions, especially those with symptoms of impaired blood flow suggesting a possible stroke (since sometimes, as with TIAs, these symptoms appear prior to a stroke). However, operations are also being done for those without symptoms but with advanced, though not severe, narrowings.

Cholesterol deposits most often occur where the internal carotid artery, supplying the brain, branches off the main (common) carotid at the middle of the neck. The normal fullness or bulge at the artery's origin is the primary site for narrowing by cholesterol, and it is readily accessible to surgery. The other branch off the common carotid artery is the external carotid, which carries blood to the face and the surface of the head (fig. 22.1).

Internal carotid narrowings cause trouble in a number of ways. It is this condition that causes TIAs, which, as mentioned in the last chapter, can cause any of the early stroke warnings and are indicators of high future stroke risk. A second result of the carotid deposits is the breaking off of cholesterol fragments or blood clots or both that are then pumped into the brain, causing small strokes. The third, often

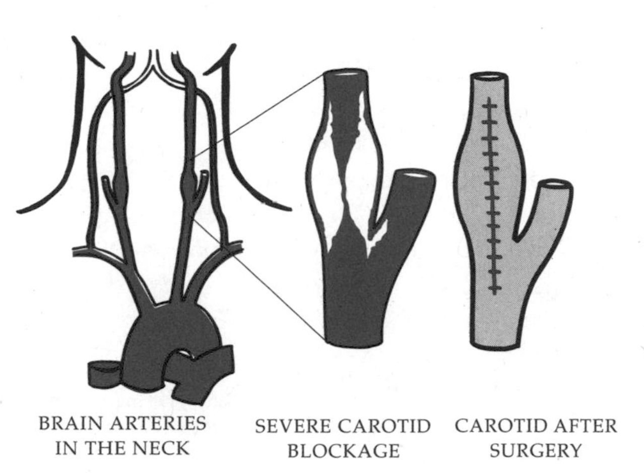

Fig. 22.1 BLOCKAGE OF BRAIN ARTERIES IN THE NECK

The larger carotid arteries nourish the upper and front parts of the brain. The more slender basilar arteries supply the bottom and rear areas. Blockage of these vessels by atherosclerosis or blood clots, or both, causes many strokes, most now preventable by removal of the cholesterol deposit through a small neck incision.

devastating, complication is complete obstruction of the internal carotid at the point of obstruction by an acute blood clot or by worsened cholesterol deposits (as shown in fig. 22.1). With this obstruction, frequently half of the body becomes totally paralyzed, and other problems also occur.

If, prior to a stroke, a stethoscope examination on the surface of the neck reveals a bruit, the doctor knows that the artery is obstructed. The next step is a sonographic (ultrasound or echo) examination, which provides a remarkably accurate outline of the cholesterol deposit. When narrowings are found and are severe, decisions about surgery are based on angiography, the X-ray procedure that uses dye injections to investigate blockages.

Neck-artery surgery consists of making a vertical slit through which the cheeselike plaque is separated from the artery wall. The deposits can be removed completely, leaving a smooth vessel wall. A temporary bypass graft is sometimes used to sustain flow during the operation, which is most often performed with the use of general anesthetic. (Some medical centers prefer to use local anesthesia.) Arteries on both sides of the neck may need surgery. If this is the case, it is accomplished at separate operations. Experienced surgeons operate with extremely low risk. However, because the use of this type of surgery is rapidly expanding, you should ask your physician to provide information about the professional records of the available surgeons in your area so that the most effective surgeon may be selected.

Surgery in patients without symptoms is under intensive investigation. Certainly, if a routine physical examination reveals the bruit in your neck and further investigation reveals severe carotid narrowing, even if you have not experienced symptoms, surgery should be considered. Remember, during your physical checkups make certain that your doctor listens to both sides of your neck with the stethoscope.

The exciting results of neck-artery surgery add another dimension to today's increasing success in preventing and treating strokes. After surgery, the blockage is not likely to return, and a repeat operation is rarely needed. Extensive investigations are being conducted to determine whether balloon angioplasty with stent insertion is as effective as this surgery. A definitive answer is not yet available.

CHAPTER 23

Hastening Recovery from a Stroke

The Role of Rehabilitation

Few illnesses interfere with daily life as much as a stroke does if it is not intercepted or treated in a timely manner. Following a debilitating stroke, the most notable problems are arm or leg paralysis (or both), speech difficulty, altered sensation all over the body, and emotional change. Taken together, the total effects of strokes in the survivors (150,000 die each year) are the leading cause of disability from all diseases in the United States. You may have experienced this problem with a parent, spouse, relative, or friend, and if you have, it has probably led you to a feeling of discouragement. All of us need to gain a better idea of what can be done for these loved ones, and we also need to remember that we ourselves might need assistance to reduce disability and improve quality of life should we have a stroke. Rehabilitation services, widely recognized to benefit many people and return them to a higher quality of life, are available in many locations and are usually reimbursed by Medicare and other third-party payers.

Most of the process of rehabilitation and returning to a happy life after a stroke can usually be directed by your personal physician, the medical professional who is already best acquainted with you physically and psychologically. The goal is to speed your return to as nearly normal functioning as possible.

If treating problems such as speech difficulty, depression, severe paralysis, and reduced bowel and bladder control is beyond the experience of a patient's personal doctor, the patient probably will be referred to a rehabilitation specialist or center, which can be very effective in assisting impaired individuals toward returning to a gainful life. This service could include physical therapy to improve the function of weakened extremities and restore mobility. If needed, speech therapy can be utilized to improve communication ability. Often, attention to depression and despondency is high on the list of needed services. Although seeing improvement in physical activity and ability to converse can lift the spirits, excellent medications also are available to further help recovering stroke sufferers through the discouragement often experienced with any serious illness—and particularly a stroke, where brain injury may contribute to the emotional change. Attention to such matters as urinary problems through urology services may mean a great deal to the patient and family, a need patients do not always voice prominently if they are embarrassed by it.

CHAPTER 24

Controlling Your Risk of a Stroke

A Summary of Dos and Don'ts

We are confronted by so many "dos and don'ts" in health care that it is easy to wind up confused and ineffective in achieving any benefit. In focusing on the broad topic of strokes, I have outlined multiple causes, effects, treatments, and preventive actions. Here, I am going to give you a compact summary of the causes of strokes and actions to take to prevent death or disability.

About 85 percent of strokes are from a cutting off or reduction of the blood supply to the brain, producing ischemia, or blood shortage. Of these strokes, 20 percent are caused by blood-clot emboli (fragments) being dislodged from the interior of the heart. Except for a very few from uncommon causes, almost all of the remaining 65 percent are caused by atherosclerosis involving arteries, from the largest down to the very smallest, that supply the brain with blood. The other 15 percent of strokes are hemorrhagic, usually from the rupture of artery aneurysms present at birth or developing later, or, less often, rupture of vessels in the congenital abnormality known as arteriovenous malformation.

The following key actions, all of which will be discussed in detail in Part V, may apply to the prevention of strokes or the prevention of serious disability from more than one type of stroke. First, elimination of cholesterol excess, the main culprit in strokes as well as in heart attacks and peripheral artery disease. (By lowering the cholesterol level, certain statin drugs can cut stroke risk by 50 percent.) Second, controlling high blood pressure, an important factor in preventing artery rupture and in controlling the development or acceleration of atherosclerosis. Third, obtaining anticoagulant treatment to prevent embolization from atrial fibrillation, a condition in which blood clots dislodge from the heart and obstruct brain arteries. Fourth, responding quickly to the early warning signs of a stroke, since early attention may mean preventing brain damage. Fifth, heeding TIAs, which are serious warnings of a possible stroke in the future, and obtaining neck-artery surgery to remove cholesterol, a highly successful procedure for avoiding future strokes. Sixth, attending to the symptoms of heart disease, especially congestive heart failure, which increases stroke risk. Seventh, women increasing their attention to the postmenopausal state, when hormone change makes increased levels of cholesterol likely. Eighth, obtaining regular physical checkups, including neck-artery examination by stethoscope, blood-pressure evaluation, and cholesterol measurements, as part of a joint commitment with your physician for long-term stroke prevention. Ninth, eliminating other cardiovascular-disease risk factors, including cigarette smoking, excess weight, and physical inactivity. And finally, applying caution when considering using highly advertised stroke-prevention products or services that promise quick health results, where the sales motivation may be financial gain to the seller rather than genuine effectiveness. Check with your doctor before buying any of these items.

As with heart disease, we have entered a new era of greatly reducing the deadly and disabling disease of stroke. Take these stroke-prevention lessons to heart!

Part V

Prevention of Heart Attacks and Strokes

Solving Problems before They Happen

CHAPTER 25

Losing Weight, Preventing Weight Gain, and How Physical Activity Benefits You

It may surprise you that rather than beginning this vital section on prevention of heart attacks and strokes with the "big three" risks (cholesterol and triglyceride excess, cigarette smoking, and hypertension), I am starting with the prevention and correction of weight excess followed by the related topic of physical inactivity. These two problems now threaten to surpass the big three in importance and may even threaten the future of the majority of Americans. So my first priority in talking about prevention is to address what you can do to lose weight to lessen your risk for heart attack and stroke.

I am not a nutritionist, but because of the significance of nutrition and diet to heart disease and stroke prevention and treatment, I have worked with nutritionists, and diet has been a primary focus of my work. I base my recommendations on decades of experience in weight control as a long-term primary-care physician to thousands of cardiovascular disease patients from a broad range of educational, economic, and geographic backgrounds, and on my continuing study of correcting the risk factor of obesity and the physical inactivity frequently associated with it.

These dual problems affect three groups in our population. The first is adults who know they have heart or blood vessel disease and may have experienced a heart attack or stroke. If you are in this group, you have a compelling, immediate need to do all you can to prevent worsening of your illness, and especially to prevent a repeat heart attack or stroke. The second group is adults who have not been diagnosed with either disease. If you are in this group, your need is to prevent the diseases' first appearance. The third group is our children. Remember, atherosclerosis, the condition that causes most heart attacks and strokes, does not begin in adulthood; it begins early in life, sometimes even in infancy.

The next seven chapters focus on diet and nutrition and how you can design a diet to reach and maintain your healthy weight and cut down on cholesterol and triglycerides. I am going to begin my discussion of creating a healthy eating plan for yourself with the evolution of my own program for weight loss and nutrition. As you will see, this program grew out of not only my patients' needs but also my own. After diet and nutrition, I will address how to create your own practical and doable exercise program, an integral part of dieting and of maintaining a healthy lifestyle.

CHAPTER 26

The Turner Weight-Loss System

The method of weight control I developed for myself and my patients grew directly out of my childhood experiences during the Great Depression. In those terrible years, there was no money for tractors or other power equipment for my family's near-bankrupt farm, so we kept it running with hard physical labor, using 3,000 to 5,000 calories daily. To prepare us for our work, my mother served a breakfast of eggs, fatback bacon, and either biscuits or pancakes, with plenty of sorghum molasses, Karo syrup, or honey. At the noon and evening meals she always had pie or cake.

As a child with these large sorts of meals, high both in carbohydrates and in calories, and a heavy work schedule on Saturdays and during the summer, I almost always became weak, shaky, and extremely hungry by midmorning and midafternoon. My mother called this the "weak trembles." I usually tried to sneak back to the house for a piece of pie or a slice of cake to relieve me. When I started college at fifteen, I weighed 135 pounds. I had not experienced abnormal weight gain because prior to college my energy expenditure had offset my large calorie and carbohydrate intake.

During college and medical school, as I grew and matured, I reached 160 pounds, but food availability was limited, and my meals were usually skimpy. However, during my hospital internship, three years of military service, and hospital residency, free food was abundant. My eating habits from childhood returned—but there was no significant physical activity to use the calories that had been consumed by farm labor. The result: by the time I returned to Springfield to practice cardiology at age twenty-eight, my weight had reached nearly 200 pounds! At first, my eating habits continued unchanged. Accustomed to sweets to relieve drops in energy, I kept small candy bars in my desk drawer to deal with the weak spells.

The shock came when, in 1947, I began to see patients with coronary disease and observed that a great many of them were overweight. Questioning them, I found that they had eating habits similar to my own. Despite my medical training, this was the first time I fully appreciated the role of high-carbohydrate intake in causing surges in insulin production by the pancreas. This in turn leads to overshooting the insulin amount needed to process ingested sugar, causing an excessive drop in blood sugar about three hours after a meal. This carbohydrate-induced drop in blood sugar, known as hypoglycemia, overstimulates the appetite. For those already eating an excessive amount of carbohydrates, this means eating more carbohydrates, resulting in excessive carbohydrate and calorie intake and weight gain.

Once I saw the eating habits my patients and I had in common, I recognized that the physiologic phenomenon of high-carbohydrate-induced hypoglycemia was stimulating our appetites and causing us to overeat. But at the time when I began my practice, authorities did not regard excess weight as a risk for heart disease, except for increasing the chances of developing diabetes.

Even by the early 1950s, when research by the American Heart Association, the U.S. government, and the pharmaceutical industry led to great strides in managing cardiovascular problems, obesity was still not highlighted in relation to heart disease. But my senior associate and I, the only cardiologists in the Southwest Missouri region, could not ignore that the high frequency of excess weight in our cardiac patients indicated that it contributed either to causing heart disease or to worsening it.

My own severe weight excess, and my experience in the military diagnosing heart attacks in young soldiers, many of whom were overweight, made me to feel that I might be the next to have a heart attack. Because of what I had observed, I knew that through my diet I could increase life expectancy, quality of life, and productivity. Thus began what amounted to what some called a crusade and others termed heart-care evangelism. This attracted so many new patients to my clinic that I wound up engaging six associates. My weight-control campaign included full care of the patient. Because there was a suggestion that cholesterol was involved in heart and blood vessel disease—although not much research had yet been done on it—I soon aimed to lower cholesterol as well as to achieve weight loss (see Chapters 27–30).

At the time I set about meeting this huge challenge of excess weight in my patients and in myself, the hospital where I worked had no diets that served my purposes, so I created my own, which the hospital soon adopted. I called these diets the Cardiac No. 1, a 1,200-calorie diet, and the Cardiac No. 2, an 1,800-calorie diet. I used the 1,200-calorie-per-day diet for average-size women and short men, who, because of their size, require fewer calories per day, and the 1,800-calorie diet for taller women and for average-size men. (See Chapter 30 for sample 1,200- and 1,800-calorie diets.) The weight-loss goal of both these plans was one pound per week.

The main item at each meal was a substantial serving of high-protein food. At breakfast, this was usually lean meat and eggs, which, with the early understanding of cholesterol's effect on heart disease, I soon changed to egg whites. With calorie limits, and an eye toward nutrition, there was no room for high-calorie items, either from fat or from unhealthy, heavily sugared carbohydrates. I have often referred to these diets as "commonsense diets."

Whether I was seeing a new patient or patients for follow-up after a heart attack or stroke, if they had excess weight I offered to work with them on dieting. Overweight patients were remarkably responsive to the opportunity. I gave each of them a diet sheet and another sheet with food caloric values. The crucial initial instruction was to avoid high-carbohydrate meals and snacks, like the ones I had been accustomed to, that were likely to induce any degree of hypoglycemic reaction.

The first big lesson I learned was that regardless of a patient's educational, economic, or geographic background, very few patients seemed willing or able to consistently follow calculated diet plans. Recognizing this early on led to what proved to be the mainstay of my long-term weight-reduction system. I stopped asking patients to follow their diet sheets to the letter. Instead, I suggested they use their diet and calorie sheets as a means of becoming familiar with caloric and carbohydrate values, so that they would have guidelines to create their own meals with varied choices each day that would produce weight loss. I stressed the importance of high-protein and low-carbohydrate breakfasts, of cutting down on fats, and of never skipping breakfast or any other meal. My revised commonsense system for dieting is simple in its approach, and in this and the next four chapters I will present it to you because, as thousands of my patients proved by putting it into practice, it works!

What I mean by "commonsense" is that my diet system is moderate, not extreme. As I will explain later in more detail, people do not follow extreme diets long-term, and often, if they start with an extreme diet, they falter in making the transition to a less extreme diet. This is why the large majority of dieters fail to keep off the weight that they may have initially lost.

A moderate diet does not take off pounds as quickly as an extreme diet does, but it is easier to follow long-term. Why? Because it is more satisfying than an extreme diet, which often leaves you feeling food deprived. A commonsense food choice system has another advantage as well: from the start it teaches you to develop and practice moderate eating habits that you will follow for the rest of your life, first to lose weight and then to maintain a healthy weight. Contrast this with an extreme diet that first leaves you feeling deprived of food and then rests on the assumption that when you reach a certain weight, you will then be able to learn and stick to moderate eating habits.

As I mentioned, I set the goal of losing one pound of fat per week. Since one pound of fat equals 3,500 calories, in order to lose one pound per week of excess weight you need to lose 500 calories of fat per day (7 days x 500 calories = 3,500 calories, or 1 pound of fat per week). This means that, on average, you need to expend 500 calories more per day than you take in.

The first step in following this plan is establishing a proper exercise program. Although I will go into further detail about this in Chapter 33, here I will share with you my observation that for the majority of people, the most attainable and sustainable form of exercise is walking. Walking expends 100 calories per mile; walking two miles per day uses 200 calories. Since your goal is to take in 500 calories per day less than you expend, if you expend 200 calories walking, this leaves 300 calories to be subtracted from your customary daily eating. Here is where the caloric value sheets play such a vital role: they help you decide which food items to eliminate and which to choose to achieve your target of taking in 500 less calories than you expend.

Among the more frequently chosen omissions in my calorie-subtraction system:

- two slices of bread (approximately 140 calories), often accomplished by skipping bread at the noon and evening meals (this works very well for me)
- one full-size pat of butter (100)
- one donut snack (200)
- one 12-ounce can of soda, containing ten teaspoons of sugar (150)
- french fries (220–440)
- fried chicken (430 calories for two pieces)
- skipping dessert (100–300) six days per week out of seven (I allowed one small piece of pie per week, and never pie à la mode)

I offered patients three key pieces of advice: First, stick to a weight-loss goal of one pound per week. Do not undertake losing two pounds per week, because the pressure would create a situation in which there would be too great a likelihood of disappointment. Second, focus on weight-loss goals for the upcoming week and month rather than on the often intimidating six-month and twelve-month weight-loss needs. And third, accept, and do not be discouraged by, occasionally failing to meet weekly expectations, and do not cancel office visits if this occurs.

Generally, at the start of a weight-loss program I saw patients once a month for a question-and-answer session. If a patient did not show the desired progress by three months or so, it was agreed that he or she would concurrently participate in Weight Watchers or TOPS (Take Off Pounds Sensibly), for the additional support offered by these organizations (see Chapter 31).

I asked patients to weigh themselves only once weekly, first thing in the morning, unclothed, after voiding, and to write the results on an index card to bring to the office on their next visit. Every twelve months I gave each patient a complete head-to-toe physical checkup, including ECG, chest X-ray, and blood and urine tests. A less complete review was conducted every six months, and at each office visit there was a brief physical examination. As patients became comfortable with their program, the length of time between office visits was extended to two months. This schedule was maintained until the individual patient's goal was reached, at which time office visits were reduced to once every three months, and later to once every six months.

Goals were set so that each person's weight would reach the target number for a normal woman or man of a particular height, regardless of the person's age (see the weight chart in Chapter 30). I do not condone stopping necessary weight loss when a person is still several pounds short of his or her goal, as some writers on diet have sanctioned. Even several pounds of excess weight increase the risk of a heart attack and stroke.

Because of the success of my weight-loss system, it received a great deal of regional media attention. Newspapers dubbed the card I asked patients to fill in with their weekly weights the "Turner Weight Watchers card," and they called my patients' agreement to work with me our "contract." The media coverage and word of mouth would have provided enough patronage to support a weight-loss clinic. But my commitment remained the treatment of cardiovascular disease patients and people seeking to avoid these diseases; I was interested in weight loss and maintenance of a healthy weight because I wanted to help patients reduce the risk of a heart attack and stroke. And this is why I am presenting my program to you. It will provide you with a strategy for planning your own weight control that you will find practical and therefore doable.

Many of my patients lost between 25 and 50 pounds, and there were a surprising number of 75- to 100-pound losers. But the only testimonial I submit for this weight-loss system is my own: applying the same principles to myself that I instilled in my patients eliminated my 40 pounds of excess weight in a year at the rate of just under one pound per week. I feel certain that this gave me a more productive and probably a longer life.

CHAPTER 27

Controlling Cholesterol, Other Blood Fats, and Triglycerides

The Role of Diet

The story of the role of diet in controlling the levels of cholesterol, other blood fats (also called lipids), and triglycerides is continuing to evolve, and you need to know about it. It provides information for understanding what makes a diet effective or ineffective for heart and blood vessel health, and thus will help you in planning your own diet. I do not want you to just take my word about why you should follow my recommendations for a diet program; I want you to *understand* why. If you understand why I am making this recommendation, it will make it easier for you to make a commitment to achieving and maintaining a healthy weight and healthy levels of cholesterol, other lipids, and triglycerides. This is a long-term commitment; in fact, it is a lifetime commitment.

Decades ago, when cholesterol's part in developing atherosclerosis became more fully appreciated and it became evident that saturated fat (animal fat) contributes to raising cholesterol, the high-fat American diet became a matter of concern. Accordingly, early recommendations by the American Heart Association for treating and preventing atherosclerosis focused primarily on dietary changes for those with heart disease. As a means of reducing elevated cholesterol levels, the AHA advised substantially reducing the consumption of total fat, especially saturated fat of animal origin, and replacing the majority of it with unsaturated fat (vegetable fat). The AHA introduced two standard diets for cholesterol reduction. They were known as Step I and Step II, and they both limited the amount of fat in the diet. This involved calculating the calories contained in fatty foods and then seeing what percentage of the total calorie intake came from these fat calories. It was a very cumbersome chore to do this.

Step I restricted total fat intake per day to 30 percent, a reduction from the usual 45 to 46 percent in the average American's diet. Saturated fat was restricted to 10 percent, down from 14 percent. The remainder of the fat content was to consist of unsaturated fats from vegetable oils. The Step II diet, for those who did not respond adequately to Step I, further restricted total fat to 20 percent and saturated fat to 7 percent.

Little was said about total calories and total carbohydrate content. Reducing fat calories increased carbohydrate intake, but as I mentioned, in these early years, contrary to my personal belief based on observation of my patients, weight excess was not considered a risk for atherosclerotic diseases except as a contributing factor to developing diabetes.

The vegetable oils initially advised (and later not recommended) were corn, sunflower, and safflower. Because these contained a number of kinds of fat, they were called polyunsaturated. Later, it was concluded that monounsaturated oils (oils containing predominantly only one kind of fat) were more beneficial, and it was advised to forego polyunsaturated oils and use only monounsaturated. Of these, canola oil became the most popular.

When the heart healthiness of people in the Mediterranean region was highlighted, experts began to recommend olive oil, another monounsaturated oil, which plays a dominant role in the Mediterranean diet. Extra virgin olive oil remains the monounsaturated oil most recommended today.

The AHA's Step I and Step II diets fell far short of expectations. Except in a few individuals, cholesterol levels dropped an average of only a few to several points, much less than needed. To help deal with this problem, in 2001 the National Cholesterol Education Program introduced the "Therapeutic Lifestyle Change Diet," which restricted fat to 30 percent of the total diet, 10 percent or less being saturated fat, and restricted protein content to 15 percent, leaving a carbohydrate content of 55 percent. The cholesterol-lowering results of this diet were also disappointing.

Remember, high-carbohydrate intake leads to hypoglycemia and stimulates the appetite, causing you to eat more. Eating an excess of carbohydrates produces more than excess weight, though; it also has another role in increasing the risk of atherosclerotic diseases. You already know that an elevated triglyceride level is a risk factor for these diseases. You may not know that triglycerides are primarily the product of carbohydrate metabolism. This means that overindulgence in carbohydrates is a primary factor in raising triglyceride levels. Thus, the subject of how much carbohydrate content should be included in the daily diet is a vital one, and I will return to it in the next chapters.

During the years of these dietary efforts to reduce cholesterol, the overweight epidemic in the United States blossomed. Today, weight excess is recognized as a risk factor for atherosclerotic diseases and is listed as a major component in metabolic syndrome, discussed in Chapter 11. Whereas in the past it was difficult to generate public interest in cholesterol reduction by diet, there was a huge public desire for weight loss, and therefore a huge market for weight-loss programs and drugs. In the following chapters, I will discuss these vital subjects. But here I want to share with you five observations on which my view of dieting for weight loss and lowering blood fat and triglyceride levels is based. I have stated some of them before, but, like the early warning signs of heart attacks and strokes, they are worth repeating because they can be lifesaving:

1. It is unreasonable to expect a short period—of weeks, months, or even a few years—of proper diet to reverse the consequences of inappropriate diet started in infancy and continued for decades.
2. Moderate diets should be started in early childhood and should be adopted by adults for the remainder of their lives, ignoring the hype and tumult of special diet promotions.
3. In formulating a moderate diet, it is unreasonable to expect people to regularly calculate the exact percentage of fats, proteins, and carbohydrates in their diet. Instead, they should have a general understanding of the proportion of these foods that should be in their diet (see Chapter 28), know which foods fall into which categories, and approximate these proportions in their daily diet.

Exact numbers do not really matter, and thinking that they do often serves as an excuse for people to abandon diets.

4. Although we must recognize the value of proper diets in stopping the inception or the worsening of cholesterol and triglyceride abnormalities, we must also recognize the limitations of diet in removing abnormalities once they are present.
5. If, as is the case with many people, diet alone does not remove cholesterol or triglyceride abnormalities, it is necessary to utilize immediately, along with diet, the advantage provided by all other types of treatment, especially cholesterol- and triglyceride-lowering drugs (see Chapter 36).

CHAPTER 28

What's Wrong with Low-Carb Diets—and What You Should Know about How Much Carbohydrates, Fat, and Protein to Include in Your Diet

In the past few years, low-carbohydrate diet plans have been extremely popular, and, indeed, have become an industry. I advocate moderate diets. Low-carbohydrate diets are not moderate diets: they lower carbohydrate intake, often to an extreme degree. Whether or not they actually say so, each low-carb diet also has its own assumptions about fat and protein intake. I disagree with the approaches of these plans. Although their popularity has begun to wane, their approach has been so pervasive, and their promise of quick weight loss so alluring, that I want you to understand exactly how these diets have been designed and what is wrong with them.

Carbohydrates, Proteins, and Fats

I am going to look briefly at carbohydrates, proteins, and fats—what they are, what foods they come from, and how our bodies process them. All of this is vital to your understanding of the low-carb diet systems and why I disagree with them.

Carbohydrates are our primary source of fuel for maintaining our body functions. Protein is the basis of the physical structure of our body other than bone. It is used to make and repair muscles, skin, ligaments, blood vessel walls, and many of the organs such as the heart, stomach, intestines, liver, and kidneys. Fat is the primary source of the blood fats (lipids) that carry nutrition throughout the body.

Carbohydrates, which consist of sugars and starches, come primarily from vegetables and grains. (It is contained in smaller amounts in nuts.) Protein comes largely from red meat, poultry, fish, egg whites, and pork. Fat comes in two forms, saturated (animal) and unsaturated (vegetable). I will discuss proteins and fats later. First, I will focus on carbohydrates.

Carbohydrates consist of sugars and starches. Sugars are sucrose (or table sugar) from sugar cane and sugar beets, fructose from fruits, and lactose from milk products. Starches come primarily from vegetables such as sweet potatoes, white potatoes, carrots, and parsnips and from grains such as beans, peas, oats, rice, wheat, and barley. Starches consist of sugars that when unprocessed are joined together and later broken down in the digestive process.

Carbohydrates are our bodies' primary source of fuel. Besides our daily intake of carbohydrates, the body supplements its needs for fuel from a carbohydrate reserve in the liver. Ingested food that we do not immediately use is stored as body fat. Fat deposits, which come not just from excess carbohydrate intake but also from excess protein and fat intake, are said to be a genetic carryover from thousands of years ago, when it was necessary to store food for use during periods of food shortages. When you overeat carbohydrates, protein, or fat, you accumulate excess body fat and thus become overweight.

Because it is critical to your understanding of low-carb diets, I am going to explain the digestion process of carbohydrates. You will recognize some of it because we have looked at it before in relation to my early eating habits.

During digestion, carbohydrates are converted in the stomach and upper intestine into glucose (simple sugars) for absorption into the bloodstream and distribution throughout the body. As glucose circulates, insulin secreted by the pancreas makes the glucose accessible to body tissues for immediate use and to the liver for storage of excess.

In their natural states, most sugars and starches from whole fruits, vegetables, and whole grains are bound together with fiber. Fiber is useful in the body, especially in bowel function, but it has no food (that is, nutritional) value. Converting carbohydrates that are combined with fiber into absorbable glucose takes longer, and is more gradual than converting sugars and starches that have been separated from fiber when they were being processed for marketing. Processed carbohydrates are rapidly broken down into glucose and quickly available for absorption in the upper intestines.

Examples of processed carbohydrates are products made from white flour such as white bread, bagels, pasta, and donuts; white rice; and fruit juice separated from fiber by squeezing. White potatoes are largely devoid of fiber in comparison with sweet potatoes.

The arrival of glucose in the bloodstream, after absorption from the upper intestine, signals the pancreas to provide insulin. When the arrival of glucose is gradual, as it is with carbohydrates that are combined with fiber, the insulin response is moderate and in keeping with the body's need. When the rise in blood glucose is more abrupt and more marked, as it is with processed carbohydrates, the production of insulin is greater and tends to overshoot the ending of glucose arrival.

This excessive duration of insulin production causes an excessive drop in the blood-glucose (or blood-sugar) level. This drop in blood sugar occurs at about three hours after the meal—and you know what happens. When blood sugar drops, it constitutes hypoglycemia, the condition I experienced during my childhood of heavy farm labor and high-carbohydrate intake. Hypoglycemia produces enormous appetite stimulation.

People with hypoglycemia are caught in a vicious circle: Excessive carbohydrate intake causes excessive insulin production, which causes a reduced blood-sugar level, which causes an increased appetite, which causes increased food intake, which results in being overweight. It also results in glucose intolerance (associated with developing prediabetes and diabetes) and other factors in metabolic syndrome.

This sequence in our ingestion and digestion of food has led to the widely publicized low-carb diets. Put in its simplest terms, severely restricting carbohydrate intake limits the appetite as well as limiting calories. It also has other important effects that I will discuss later and contribute to my disagreement with these diets.

Looking at Four Low-Carb Diets

The first publicly marketed, extremely low-carbohydrate program was the Atkins plan, introduced in 1972 by Dr. Robert C. Atkins in his book *The Atkins Diet Revolution.*[1] It called for no restriction of fat content or of fat type, and was severely criticized by the medical community because it sanctioned unlimited consumption of saturated fats, already known to be a high risk for coronary artery and other atherosclerotic diseases.

After Atkins's death, a revised edition, *Atkins for Life,* was published in May 2004.[2] This revised plan advocates inclusion of monounsaturated fats but persists in the sanction of saturated fats, so in addition to being a low-carb diet, the Atkins diet might also be called a high-fat diet.

Drs. Michael and Mary Dan Eades introduced the "Protein Power Diet" in their book *Protein Power.*[3] The Protein Power Diet has three phases during all of which carbohydrate intake is restricted to varying degrees of severity. The first two phases allow less carbohydrate intake than is permitted in a strict diabetic diet, in which, because of problems with insulin production, carbohydrates are of necessity restricted to a minimum. The third phase gradually increases protein intake, and it increases carbohydrate intake to about 100 grams, similar to the amount specified in extremely strict diabetic diets.

Fat consumption is unlimited, with emphasis on monounsaturated fats, chiefly olive oil. The book gives detailed information about hormonal and other factors concerned with food utilization, but no data are provided on average rates of weight loss, length of time required to achieve weight-loss goals, or the percentage of people who comply with the program long-term.

The South Beach Diet was introduced in 2003 with a book by cardiologist Arthur Agatston.[4] Despite Agatston's opening statement that "the South Beach diet is not low-carb," the diet restricts carbohydrate intake to varying degrees of severity. This diet, too, consists of three phases. An initial quick weight-loss stage, Phase One, lasts two weeks or slightly more; Phase Two, longer-term weight reduction, lasts up to a year or longer, until the weight-reduction goal is reached; and Phase Three is the long-term maintenance phase.

Agatston states that the program is not concerned with calories or related proportions of carbohydrates, proteins, or fats. However, as I mentioned, the plan does focus on carbohydrate restriction; it is extremely strict in Phase One, somewhat less strict in Phase Two, and less strict but still limited in Phase Three.

Dr. Fred Pescatore introduced another low-carb plan, the Hamptons Diet, in 2004.[5] Pescatore states that earlier in his career he was associate medical director of the Atkins Agency in New York. While there, he began to disagree with Atkins's policy that "all fats are good fats," and he left his post.

In *The Hamptons Diet,* published after Atkins's death, Pescatore sets forth his opposing view: that the dietary saturated fat sanctioned by Atkins should be replaced by monounsaturated fats, to the greatest extent possible. Pescatore describes his program as "a modified low-carb approach." He says patients can achieve up to fourteen pounds of weight loss in the first fourteen days. The diet's cornerstones are carbohydrate restriction and the use of macadamia oil as the primary monounsaturated oil.

Like the previously discussed low-carb diets, the Hamptons Diet also has three phases, during all of which carbohydrate intake is severely restricted to less grams per day than is prescribed in extremely strict diabetic diets.

Although some of the information conveyed along with these low-carb diet plans has value—Pescatore presents a good case for macadamia-nut oil, for example, which he says has 30 percent more unsaturates than olive oil—I strongly disagree with their overall approaches. Here is a point-by-point list of my comments about and disagreements with these programs. First, all low-carb diets have an initial phase of two to four weeks or longer during which the carbohydrate intake is profoundly reduced to less than 120 calories, or 30 grams, per day. You could consume this much by drinking a 1-cup-size bottle or can of unsweetened apple juice (117 calories). Second, program creators emphasize the rapid weight loss that occurs during the induction phase of their programs, but none reports that this loss is mainly water, not fat, and that it results from ketosis, the process that is induced by carbohydrate restriction and causes increased urine output (see Chapter 26). This is important information to leave out, because ketosis may result in an undesirable state of dehydration. In writing about the two-week start-up phase of the South Beach Diet, Agatston, for example, repeatedly states that during the first two weeks those who follow his program will lose between eight and thirteen pounds. He makes no mention of the fact that this is not fat loss but fluid loss resulting from ketosis. Third, program creators also do not discuss the fact that ketosis may continue into their programs' later phases, even though carbohydrate allowances are somewhat increased. There are strong disagreements in the medical community concerning whether there are harmful effects from long-term ketosis. Fourth, low-carb programs give insufficient specifics regarding calorie control. Fifth, the relative proportions of carbohydrates, protein, and fat contained in these programs are at odds with the most recent scientific recommendations (I will provide these for you at the end of this chapter). Sixth, there is no emphasis in these diet programs on allying yourself with a personal physician early in the course of dealing with the lifelong health issue of excess weight. Indeed, the books promoting these low-carbohydrate programs seem to promote a "do-it-yourself" philosophy. Similarly, they do not recommend joining a reputable weight-loss organization. Seventh, exercise recommendations vary widely in degree of emphasis, type, and duration. Types of exercise include walking, jogging, and weight lifting, without relating these choices to physical capability. Not all of these programs adequately detail the relationship between exercise and expenditure of calories and the degree of weight loss. Suggested durations range from twenty to thirty minutes twice weekly, to one hour per day, to no exercise at all (the South Beach Diet says it can accomplish weight-loss goals with or without exercise). Eighth, all the programs provide an abundance of meal plans and recipes prepared by dieticians, chefs, and restaurateurs. Many of these recipes are elaborate, and some would require a chef to follow them. I question how many of you would have the time or inclination to prepare these year-round, year after year. Finally, the program creators do not give sufficient indication of the long-term effectiveness of their plans. The numerous testimonials they provide do not give this information. It is my opinion that these programs are so restrictive of carbohydrates and so complicated to follow that most people will be unable to comply with them long-term, let alone for the rest of their lives.

Now that I have told you my objections to low-carb diets, I am going to present you with diet guidelines, based on scientific studies, which will give you the information you need to create your own healthy weight-loss or weight-maintenance diet.

What Research Recommends about Carbohydrates, Proteins, and Fats in the Daily Diet

In 2004 Ronald M. Krauss, M.D., an adjunct professor of nutrition at the University of California at Berkeley and dietary consultant to the American Heart Association, gave an interview that provides a national overview of reduced-carbohydrate diets and weight control.[6] In the interview, Krauss discussed the report he delivered at the annual AHA meeting, which focused on the effects of low-carb diets on the blood-fat abnormalities that generate atherosclerosis. Krauss is one of our nation's foremost experts on nutrition. I am summarizing his report for two reasons. The first is that he analyzes low-carb diets; the second, and more important, reason is that the report presents vital information, based on respected research, about how you should think about the proportions of carbohydrates, fats, and protein in your diet.

The analysis begins with a look back at the National Cholesterol Education Plan's 2001 diet mentioned in the previous chapter. This diet recommended a carbohydrate intake of 55 percent, a number that since then has been greatly criticized as too high both for weight loss and for the reduction of cholesterol, other blood fats, and triglycerides. The data showed that when calories were left unchanged and carbohydrates were reduced in steps from the NCEP's 55 percent to 40 percent, fat was left at 30 percent, and protein was increased from 15 to 30 percent, there was a significant improvement of abnormal lipid patterns. The report also showed that adding a weight-reduction component to the program by cutting total calories further lowered lipid levels and resulted in a twelve-pound average loss of weight in nine weeks.

The carbohydrate reductions in these studies were far less than the extreme reductions in the initial phases of low-carbohydrate diet plans. The report emphasizes that with calorie control, weight loss does not depend on whether the diets are low carb, high carb, low fat, or high fat. The vital factor for weight loss is reducing the number of calories consumed.

Krauss states that until we have evidence that any of these more extreme diets are effective and safe over the long-term, we cannot recommend them as the answer. The data show that although these diets do help people get off to a quick start in weight loss, over the course of time—and certainly after six months—there is a progressive falling off of benefits from these extreme diets because people abandon them. Krauss emphasizes that more moderate diets can be sustained long-term and urges including abundant exercise. He also urges the continuing, active participation of your physician in your progress. As you know, this concurs with my experience in achieving effective weight loss for my patients and for myself, and with my recommendations for you.

I mentioned Krauss's observation that the early stages of low-carb diets are far more restrictive than the 40 percent daily carbohydrate intake his studies recommend. The following shows a comparison of the report's recommendations for carbohydrate intake to those of a low-carb diet to see how they would translate in your daily diet:

> Let's look at the maintenance diet of a 5′4″ woman who weighs 120 pounds, the weight that is considered normal and healthy for a woman her size. In order for her to maintain this weight—without losing or gaining weight—her total calorie requirement per day is 1,560. Carbohydrates have approximately 4 calories per gram. Thus, in a 1,560-calorie-per-day diet, meeting Krauss's recommended carbohydrate intake of 40 percent means eating 624 calories, or 156 grams, of carbohydrates per day (40 percent of 1,560 calories = 624 calories = 156 grams).
>
> If you had the same caloric intake needs as the woman in our example, the carbohydrate content of your three meals on any given day could include one small apple (80 calories), half a cup of cooked oatmeal (73.5), one-half of a pink grapefruit (52), one piece of whole-wheat toast (69), an ear of corn (172), half a cup of raspberries (32), and a moderate-size baked sweet potato or white potato (about 145).
>
> Now let's look at the carbohydrates permitted by one of the low-carb diets. During its start-up phase, the Hamptons Diet restricts carbohydrates to a maximum of 120 calories, or 30 grams, at most. This is less than 8 percent of an average woman's total daily 1,560 calorie intake—about 20 percent of the carbohydrate intake Krauss's report recommends. In terms of food, this would mean if the carbohydrate content of your three meals on any given day included one small apple (80 calories) and one-half of a pink grapefruit (52), you would be exceeding the prescribed carbohydrate intake by 12 calories, or 3 grams.
>
> For men, whose calorie counts are far higher and for whom the Hamptons Diet prescribes the same 120 calories, or 30 grams, of carbohydrates, the differences during the first phase are even more marked.
>
> The Hamptons Diet also restricts carbohydrate intake in its next two phases to far less than the 40 percent that Krauss recommends. Even the third phase, the maintenance phase, during which food consumption goes up, advises a daily carbohydrate intake of only

17 percent for both men and women, less than half of Krauss's 40 percent.

The above example shows what makes low-carb diets extreme, and their extremeness is what makes them difficult to follow long-term. By contrast, the ratio of 30 percent protein, 40 percent carbohydrate, and 30 percent fat that Krauss recommends is reasonable for a daily diet and attainable for a lifetime. This ratio of proteins, carbohydrates, and fats is successful in lowering abnormal blood-lipid levels and, therefore, is also effective in maintaining healthy lipid levels.

At the end of the interview, Krauss concludes, "We are facing a blitz of promotional literature that I think is confusing the public. . . . We've seen such a success of these [low-carb] diets . . . because of the very compelling marketing tools that are used to promote [them]. I feel that the word of science and reason gets lost in all that tremendous amount of noise." Take away the noise and you are left with the cardinal fact of weight control: *Weight excess does not occur unless calorie intake exceeds calorie expenditure. This means that weight loss cannot occur without reducing calorie intake below calorie expenditure.*

It is important to remember that because weight loss does depend on calorie intake being less than calorie expenditure and not on the relative amounts of fat, carbohydrate, and protein in the diet, this does not imply that an unlimited amount of fat is permissible. I am repeating this because the average diet in our country contains a tremendous amount of fat. In fact, the AHA estimates that in the average American diet, the total amount of saturated fat is 46 percent! That is almost *half* of the average daily diet! And it is not even *total* fat content, because it does not include polyunsaturated fats from vegetables, the healthier fats. There is no question that people must restrict saturated fats. Because saturated fats are high in calories, reducing your intake of these fats is essential to losing weight. Once again, this means that a moderate diet program that combines Krauss's guidelines with moderate calorie reduction serves the dual objective of weight control and, by lowering unhealthy blood-fat levels, reducing the risk of heart disease and strokes.

There is another fact about fats that is rarely mentioned by promoters of popular diet plans but that you must be aware of in order to lose weight. Notwithstanding general agreement that replacing the majority of saturated fat in your diet with monounsaturated fat reduces heart risk, an excess amount of monounsaturated fats can be as fattening as calories from any other source. Olive oil contains 120 calories per tablespoon, as does macadamia-nut oil, Pescatore's recommendation. Therefore, consuming large amounts of monounsaturated oil—say, three tablespoons of olive oil on your salads and vegetables—will put weight on rather than take it off.

Once again, I recommend these guidelines for your daily diet: 30 percent protein, 40 percent carbohydrates, and 30 percent fat, with most fat being monounsaturated. And if you are on a weight-loss or weight-maintenance diet, keep in mind that every tablespoon of monounsaturated fat contains 120 calories and that you have to take these calories into consideration in order to reach your total calorie target for that day. I am not telling you that you have to go around with a calculator figuring out calories and exact proportions of proteins, carbohydrates, and fats. My main objective is for you to have a diet that is practical and doable on a long-term basis. By learning about nutrition and your target weight goal, and by familiarizing yourself with the sample diets and calorie chart I provide for you in Chapter 30, you will find that soon you will be able to make approximations and estimates almost automatically. Inevitably, your food choices will vary from day to day, but as you become familiar with the approximate caloric and cholesterol content of different foods (high, moderate, or low?), you will be able to make choices of what to include in each meal. I want dieting to be as easy for you as possible.

That is why I am not just giving you a diet to follow; I am explaining to you the whys behind creating a moderate diet, and showing you how to tailor a diet to your specific needs and tastes. I want to teach you how to come up with a diet plan that will allow you some spontaneity, thus helping you to feel satisfied rather than deprived. In my experience this is the only kind of plan that works long-term—indeed, lifelong.

CHAPTER 29

Tips for Weight Loss, Weight Maintenance, and Lowering Cholesterol

You now know that your weight-loss and cholesterol-lowering diet should include 30 percent protein, 40 percent carbohydrates, and 30 percent fat. And you know that once you have achieved your targets, your maintenance diet should include the same proportions. But what foods should you eat to meet your targets? And what foods should you exclude? In this chapter, I will talk about food choices and give you tips for planning breakfasts, lunches, and dinners. Along with the information you have already gotten, this will give you the background you need to use the charts and sample weight-loss diets in the next chapter to create your own diet.

Remember, my goal is for you to be able to follow the diet you create for a lifetime. It will not be a rigid system that you must follow to the letter and would therefore be likely to abandon within months. Instead, it will be a moderate diet, a new way of eating and of thinking about food that will help you make appropriate choices at every meal, choices that will benefit your heart health, your blood vessel health, and your overall health.

Tips for Increasing Monounsaturated Fat and Cutting Down on Saturated Fat

Fat, regardless of type (saturated or unsaturated), has 2.25 times the number of calories as the same amount of pure sugar. Right now, most of your fat intake is probably of saturated fat from animals. Remember that since saturated fat is less healthy for your blood vessels and heart, cutting down on animal fat will help you achieve two things simultaneously: it will reduce calories, and it will reduce your risk of a heart attack and stroke.

You already know that most of the 30 percent of fat included in your diet should come from monounsaturated fats such as olive oil or, as Pescatore recommends, macadamia-nut oil (especially for cooking). In moderate amounts, these oils can be used on salads and vegetables. Since they have 120 calories per tablespoon, two tablespoons contain 240 calories.

If you are an average-size woman on a 1,200-calorie-per-day weight-loss diet, your goal is to take in 360 calories per day from fats (30 percent of 1,200 = 360). So two tablespoons of a monounsaturated oil per day gives you two-thirds of your daily fat requirement in a healthy form. If you are a woman or a man of about 5′6″ on an 1,800-calorie-per-day weight-loss diet, your goal is to take in 540 calories per day from fats (30 percent of 1,800 = 540). So the 240 calories contained in two tablespoons of a monounsaturated oil gives you almost half of your daily fat requirement.

The following are tips my patients found helpful and easy to put into practice to reduce the amount of saturated fat in meals:

- Omit cream and half-and-half from your diet.
- Change from whole milk to skim milk or 1 percent butterfat milk. (Stirring in two heaping tablespoons of skim milk powder, which is pure protein, into a quart of skim milk improves the taste).
- Reduce the amount of butter at the table. A large pat of butter contains 100 calories, 8 percent of your total calorie intake for a day if you are on a 1,200-calorie weight-loss diet and more than one-quarter of your total daily fat allowance if you are following the 30/40/30 recommendation.
- In cutting down on butter, do not use any hydrogenated products. Hydrogenation is the process that converts liquid vegetable fats to solids and was widely used in preparing hard-stick margarine until it was discovered that it produced a harmful substance known as transfat (an intermediate phase in the hardening process of converting vegetable fat into satu-

rated fat). You should omit all spreads that do not clearly state that hydrogenation is not involved in their manufacture. Be aware that hydrogenation is also used extensively to give texture to processed foods. Check all labels of processed foods to make certain that hydrogenation is not involved.

- Switch from high-butterfat ice creams to sherbets and low-fat preparations (soy "ice cream" has less fat, for example).
- Discard all egg yolks (put them down the drain!). Advertising to the contrary, there is no proven "safe" egg yolk cholesterol. Here's why: Egg yolk cholesterol is a portion of the total fat content in a diet. The American Heart Association advocates restricting oral cholesterol intake to 300 milligrams per day at most and ideally to 200. One large whole egg contains 211 milligrams of cholesterol or more. So by eating one egg yolk, you are exceeding the AHA's ideal daily amount of 200 milligrams of cholesterol. In view of the proven role of cholesterol in causing atherosclerosis, it makes no sense to eat egg yolks.
- Omit *all* deep-fried foods from your diet. You have heard this for years, and it is true.
- Trim all visible fat from meat, and remove the skin from chicken and other poultry before cooking.
- Omit all hot dogs and luncheon meats from your diet unless they are certified to have been prepared from pure lean beef. (Most hot dogs should be considered as fat sources, not high-protein foods.)
- With regret, because I used to like it so much, I advise that you omit bacon from your diet. Bacon is predominantly fat.
- Liver, sweetbreads, and kidney should also be omitted.
- In all meals, especially breakfast, include main courses consisting of high-protein foods.

Tips for Including Protein in Your Diet while Cutting Down on Saturated Fats

I have advised you to include servings of high-protein foods in each meal. Since protein often comes from meat and, therefore, is often accompanied by saturated fat, you may be wondering how you can include protein in every meal and still cut down on saturated fat.

First, I want to remind you that Krauss says *most* fat in your diet should be monounsaturated; by most, he means the large majority of it. A small amount of saturated fats in lean meats is acceptable (and, in fact, research is being done to see whether including some saturated fat in your diet may have a beneficial effect in lessening the amount of small, dense particles in LDL cholesterol).

Chicken and turkey are splendid protein sources. Authorities favor white meat because it is leaner. An easy way of getting white meat is buying only chicken and turkey breasts. If you prefer the whole chicken or turkey, discard the livers but do not throw away the thighs and legs. Broil or bake them with the skin and fat removed. Baking a large turkey breast will supply lunch and dinner protein for several meals. Ground white meat turkey or chicken makes great burgers or turkey or chicken loaf.

Lean beef and lamb, with fat trimmed off, are excellent protein sources. As long as you trim away fat, less concern is expressed about the moderate fat marbling of better cuts of red meat since the primary issue is its high-protein content.

If you ask at the butcher counter, supermarkets will generally prepare sliced-beef "breakfast steaks" (small, thin pieces) that cook quickly, or you can buy larger pieces and cut breakfast steaks yourself.

Some people do not include pork in their diets, but for those of you who do, lean pork with the fat trimmed off is also an excellent source of protein. It should be cooked well to eliminate the risk of trichinosis in uncooked pork. For those who eat pork, Canadian bacon is very lean and an excellent source of breakfast protein.

What about fish as a source of protein? The AHA has recommended two servings a week of fatty fish because of its high omega-3 fatty-acid content. (Omega 3, a component of certain fats found in some fish, certain nuts, and other foods, is beneficial in lipid control.) Currently, however, the levels of mercury, methylmercury, PCBs (polychlorinated biphenyls), and other toxins in many fish have caused concern. Some fish are less contaminated than others, and a few varieties are considered safe to eat in moderate amounts. Among factors that affect contamination are the purity of the body of water in which the fish is raised, the size of the fish (large fish are more contaminated), and the life span of the fish (those that live longer accumulate more mercury). Some writers on nutrition have also raised concerns about antibiotics used in farm-raised fish. For most adults, two moderate servings of the safest fish available in your area seems acceptable. You can get recommendations for fish safety and consumption by checking the U.S. Food and Drug Administration (FDA) and U.S. Environmental Protection Agency (EPA) reports, as well as by state agencies, readily available on the Internet. Pregnant women and women who plan to be pregnant must check to see which fish and in what amounts are acceptable for them. Parents must also be careful about fish in their young children's diets. Check FDA and EPA guidelines to see what kinds of fish and in what serving amounts are acceptable for young children. Capsules of omega 3 are available and are currently advised by many as an addition to your diet.

Egg whites are an excellent, economical protein source. Two or three whites of eggs, cooked with lean meat, can be your staple breakfast.

Cottage cheese is a neglected protein source. Low-fat cottage cheese is available, but switching from half a cup of regular cottage cheese to half a cup of low-fat reduces fat calories by only 40 and fat grams by 4.5. This means the advantage of choosing the low-fat variety, which many people find unpalatable, provides only a limited advantage. If you prefer the taste of regular cottage cheese, it may not be worth switching to low-calorie cottage cheese for the fat calories you would save, as long as you are sufficiently limiting your intake of other fats. Be aware that some people are allergic to dairy products such as milk and cheeses. Fortunately, a range of products made from soy or rice milk can be substituted. They are generally lower in fat—but check labels for calories and protein and fat contents.

Other types of cheese are also important protein sources. A number of reduced-fat versions are available, but, again, if you prefer the taste of regular cheese of a particular variety, compare the fat calories in both types to see if the switch to the lower-calorie kind is justified. For example, switching from a 1-ounce (30 gram) serving of regular mozzarella to the same size serving of low-fat mozzarella reduces fat calories by 30 (about 3 grams). Since cheeses vary in fat content, you have to compare fat contents of the regular and low-fat varieties one cheese at a time in order to make an appropriate choice.

Beans of all kinds have a high protein content. Soybean products, commonly called soy, are 40 to 50 percent protein. In the past, they were generally considered to significantly reduce LDL cholesterol if eaten in sufficient quantity. However, in 2006 the AHA reported new studies that showed soy's effect on LDL cholesterol reduction to average only 3 percent. Consequently, the AHA advised that soy not be consumed for the purpose of cholesterol reduction.

Another source of protein is peanut butter. Peanuts are not nuts, but legumes. The polyunsaturated fat in peanut oil is not equal to the monounsaturated fat of olive oil or nut oils such as macadamia oil, but on occasion, peanut butter, in a small amount, may offer a handy way to provide a quick breakfast protein, especially for children. Check the label on peanut butter to make sure that no hydrogenated or saturated fat has been added in processing. *And make sure you are not allergic to peanuts, since consuming peanuts in any form can be lethal to those who are allergic to them.*

Tips for Choosing Carbohydrates in Your Diet

Just how good are "good carbs"? How bad are "bad carbs"? And what do you have to know about "good carbs" and "bad carbs" to make the right choices for your diet? Those carbohydrates (sugars and starches) that are considered "good" exist in close association with fiber. These include whole grains (grains that are unprocessed), vegetables, and most fruits. The fiber slows digestion. As a result, when intake of "good" carbs is moderate, the rise in insulin is gradual and moderate, and blood sugar returns to a normal level after the glucose produced from these carbs is absorbed into the bloodstream. "Bad carbs" are those that have been separated from fiber in processing or refining, and those that occur naturally without fiber, such as white potatoes.

Refined carbohydrates include table sugar (sucrose), sugar syrups, juices squeezed from fruits, cereals, jams and jellies, candies, products made from white flour (white bread, buns, bagels, pastries, donuts, cookies, pasta, pretzels, hot cakes, and waffles), and processed grains (such as white rice or instant hot cereals). These, and white potatoes, are more rapidly digested and absorbed, causing a sharp and more marked increase in insulin that may overshoot the completion of the processing of the carbohydrate, leading to a fall in blood sugar to below-normal levels. This is hypoglycemia, which stimulates the appetite, causing excess food intake and weight gain.

Besides containing fiber, there is another advantage of "good carbs" that you should know about: research shows that whole grains, a primary source of "good carbs," contain antioxidants (agents that interfere with the oxidizing of cholesterol into a form that enables it to attach to artery walls). Whole grains also contain other substances that are beneficial for reducing the risk of cancer and coronary disease. These antioxidants and other substances are removed during the processing of "bad carbs."

In making your food choices for your diet—especially if the goal is weight loss—there are a few other things you need to know about "good carbs" versus "bad." It is vital to recognize that eating *too many* good carbs causes hypoglycemia just as eating too many bad carbs will; in other words, the *amount* of carbs you eat is the crucial factor in terms of hypoglycemia. "Good carbs" also generally contain as many calories as "bad carbs." Since being overweight is one of the major risk factors, you cannot go hog wild eating good carbs.

So although you should not overindulge in "good carbs," they have the advantages of being digested more gradually, helping bowel function, and, in the case of whole grains, adding substances to the diet that will improve overall health. Does this mean that you can never eat a white potato? Or that a small portion of white rice rather than brown is terrible for you? No—but it is wise to combine it in a meal with green leafy vegetables as you appropriately cater to your tastes. And when you can, have "good carbs"—and, again, eat them in small portions.

Including Vegetables, Fruit, and Nuts in Your Diet

Farm-fresh vegetables and fruits provide many nutrients, including a full range of vitamins (except B_{12}, which comes mainly from meat) and folic acid. Besides also giving us starches and sugars, they, like whole grains, provide the fiber essential to our diets. (Be aware that storage and processing dilute or destroy nutrients, so canned, frozen, or any other kind of packaged and prepared vegetable or fruit is never preferable to fresh produce.)

As you will see, among my meal-planning tips is that every lunch and dinner should contain vegetables and fruit, farm fresh whenever possible. Breakfasts can include fruits or vegetables as well.

Green leafy vegetables are particularly low in calories and therefore are wonderful to include in a weight-loss or weight-maintenance diet (see the calorie chart in the next chapter).

- Depending on the variety, a head of lettuce has only 29 to 65 calories.
- 1 cup of cooked fresh spinach has 8 to 10 calories.
- 1 cup of cooked fresh kale has 36 calories.
- 1 cup of cooked fresh Swiss chard has 35 calories.
- Sweet and white potatoes, starchier vegetables, are higher in calories, but if servings are moderate, neither is extraordinarily high. A white potato of moderate size has about 145 calories; a cooked sweet potato of moderate size has the same or less.

Some fruits, like blueberries (1 cup = 83 calories), are lower in calories than others, like mangos (medium size = 135).

As mentioned, nuts are a source of protein and, like macadamia nuts, also a source of certain oils. Recognize, however, that many people are allergic to nuts (and also, as mentioned, legumes such as peanuts). Therefore, nuts and peanuts are not an appropriate part of every diet. Nuts are also not low in calories. For example, ¼ cup of unsalted almonds contains 206 calories, ¼ cup of walnuts contains 163, and ¼ cup of unsalted cashews contains 320. If you are not allergic to nuts and include them in your diet as a snack food, eat them sparingly in the amounts suggested in the sample diets in Chapter 30, and always eat them unsalted in order to not adversely affect your blood pressure (see Chapter 39). Be aware as well that some experts on nutrition are advising that raw nuts are healthier than roasted.

Organic Foods

Today in many communities, organic foods are available in health food stores, health food supermarkets, organic sections of regular supermarkets, and at farm stands or farmers' markets. In some communities, they may be bought on the Internet and delivered to your door (in New York, for example, a full range of organic foods for delivery may be ordered online at http://www.FreshDirect.com).

Certified organic vegetables, fruits, grains, and nuts are grown without the use of pesticides or chemical fertilizers, and they are not processed. Although organic foods are not directly related to weight control or cholesterol reduction, some people prefer them because they are often tastier and because of the perception that they are healthier. Organic vegetables and fruits are also farm fresh and therefore contain more nutrients than nonorganic or processed vegetables and fruits. Certified organic red meats, poultry, and eggs contain no hormones, antibiotics, or other chemicals that have been injected or added to the animals' feed.

There are more stringent guidelines for organic foods that differentiate them from foods that are called "natural" that meet certain of these guidelines but not others. Genuine organic food is always certified organic.

Organic foods are generally more expensive. If they are available in your community, research and decide about the benefits of each kind, and see which ones you feel may be important to include in your diet.

Tips for Planning Breakfasts, Lunches, and Dinners

The following dietary pointers are based on all the nutritional and diet information I have presented. First, don't skip breakfast! You have always heard it is the most important meal of the day, and it is. A healthy, satisfying breakfast will prevent the escalation of your appetite as the day progresses.

Your breakfast should include at least one serving of protein and one whole-grain carbohydrate. Eliminate the cold-cereal-and-orange-juice-on-the-run breakfast. Cold cereals are mainly processed carbohydrates. "High-protein" cereal is a misnomer—there is no such thing as a truly high-protein cereal. Most orange juice is no more than diluted, high-calorie sugar syrup with flavoring and vitamin C added.

If you have a slice of bread as your whole-grain carbohydrate, choose whole wheat. If you are allergic to wheat, choose another whole-grain bread, and limit it to one slice. Whole-grain oat or oat-bran cereal is a great alternative to a slice of bread and will help lower your cholesterol. Steel-cut oats (a whole, unprocessed grain) are available in many supermarkets as well as health food stores. I do not recommend including oat or oat-bran cereal in a *weight-loss* diet. In a weight-maintenance diet, remember to serve yourself only a small (or at most moderate) portion of oatmeal or oat bran, since you do not want to consume too many calories even from good carbs. Other whole-grain cereals to choose from are rye, quinoa, barley, kamut, millet, and spelt (brown rice is also a whole grain and may be used as a hot breakfast cereal). You may not have made these cereals before, but they are easy to prepare, and cooking instructions, along with calories, are on the packages. Again, do not include cereals in a weight-loss diet, and in a maintenance diet, make sure cereal portions are small to moderate in size.

Egg whites or Egg Beaters make a great protein serving, as does a thin precut breakfast steak or a small portion of skinless white chicken or turkey breast (baked or broiled, which can be done beforehand). These options make a great breakfast served with a slice of whole-grain bread and a vegetable or piece of fruit.

Skip the bacon. Remember, it is more fat than protein.

As mentioned, whole fresh fruit or canned fruit (without sugar) is a good addition to your breakfast. But remember the centerpiece of breakfast must be a whole-grain carbohydrate and a protein.

A green leafy vegetable, such as spinach or kale, can be a good addition to your breakfast. Two or three slices of tomato are also a good accompaniment to egg whites or a breakfast steak and whole-grain bread.

Eliminate sugar in beverages and in cooked cereals. If you need a bit of sweetener in cooked cereals, use a small amount of unprocessed fruit juice, a small amount of unsweetened applesauce, or a small amount of artificial sweetener.

Save pancakes or waffles with a small amount of syrup for very special, rare occasions. They will likely cause hypoglycemia at three hours, forcing you to eat again.

Based on the same principles, here are pointers for lunches, snacks, and dinners. Like breakfasts, lunches and dinners should include one moderate-size serving of protein and one moderate-size serving of carbohydrates. They should also include green leafy vegetables and fresh or sugar-free canned fruits.

To cut down on calories, omit bread from your lunches and dinners. If you are on a weight-loss diet and you want a slice of whole-grain bread at lunch, eliminate all other lunch carbohydrates.

Salads with protein (like white-meat turkey or chicken, lean beef, or, twice per week, a healthy fish), dressed with one tablespoon or less of olive oil (or another monounsaturated oil) and lemon or vinegar, make filling, nutritious, low-calorie lunches. Since the caloric content of lettuce and other green leafy vegetables is so low, your salad can be quite large as long as the serving of protein is moderate in size.

Some diet plans call for midmorning and midafternoon snacks that, if improperly chosen, can add undesirable calories. With reasonable attention to moderation of carbohydrates at mealtimes, you will not have the three-hour appetite surge from a blood-sugar drop. A moderately low-calorie, low-carbohydrate fruit such as an apple or a calorie-free beverage such as herbal tea is a better choice for a snack. Or you can have a small green salad with dressing.

Skip the donuts. One uncoated donut per day will add one pound to your weight per month, twelve pounds in a year. One of the fancier kinds of donuts per day, at 200 calories each, will put on a pound in less than three weeks.

Potato chips are tempting but hazardous. They are high in both carbohydrate and fat. One large chip may contain ten calories—and, as the commercial used to say, "Bet you can't eat just one!"

As with breakfast, eliminate sugar from all beverages and all cooking. Use unsweetened drinks like mineral water or flat water rather than sweetened drinks. If you crave fruit juices, check the calorie count of unprocessed fruit juices such as apple juice and allow yourself a moderate amount. You can also dilute fruit juices with water to lower the number of calories while retaining the taste you enjoy. If you choose to include artificial sweeteners in your diet, artificially sweetened sodas save you 150 calories per 12-ounce can over sodas containing sugar, but make sure to drink them in moderation.

As mentioned, your dinner should include one moderate serving of protein (lean beef or lamb, chicken or turkey with the skin removed, and a healthy fish twice a week), one moderate serving of carbohydrates (sweet or white potatoes, brown rice, or millet), and green leafy vegetables. The same principle that makes a large salad good for lunch makes large portions of green leafy vegetables work well as part of your dinner. They are nutritious, filling, and low in calories. Steamed, with less than a teaspoon of olive oil sprinkled after cooking, they are extremely tasty.

Contrary to what some diet writers are saying, white potatoes, as I have mentioned, especially when eaten in moderation and at the same time as other vegetables, are acceptable and will not cause between-meal appetite stimulation. Some people are born with a tendency toward more brisk insulin responses to carbohydrates, but this should present no problem when eating a moderate-size portion of white potatoes.

For dessert, have a piece of fruit or an unsweetened or naturally sweetened fruit dessert. An apple baked in a small amount of diluted unsweetened apple juice has less than 125 calories. A half-cup of unsweetened applesauce has 50 to 100 calories, depending on its preparation (read the label on the jar or can for number of calories in a specific applesauce).

Reduce higher-calorie desserts to one per week at your "special meal." Review the calorie values of these desserts in the next chapter to make sure they are not unreasonable. For your once-a-week special meal, it is all right to go over your daily average by 100 to 200 calories, which you can easily take off when you resume your diet. For example, I allow myself a small piece of pumpkin pie but not apple pie à la mode, which was previously my favorite.

Tips for Dining in Restaurants

From time to time, most people eat in restaurants as part of their business and social lives. Many people use eating in restaurants as an excuse to regularly go off their diets. The results? Weight gain, frustration, and, often, a depressed feeling that you are never going to achieve your weight-loss goals. With the following in mind, you can enjoy eating in restaurants and remain on-track with your diet.

- Only eat in those restaurants that are happy to cater to your wishes.
- Do not hesitate to make your wishes known. Be sure to tell the server clearly exactly what you want and do not want in the preparation of your meal.
- Skip the bread. Sending back the basket untouched removes temptation.

* A low-calorie salad or soup will take the edge off your appetite. Be aware that many salad dressings are extremely high in calories and cholesterol. For a healthy, lower-calorie choice, ask for olive oil and lemon to be served on the side.
* All sauces should be eliminated from meats and vegetables. Grilled meat is delicious, as are steamed vegetables. Olive oil (in a small amount), herbs, spices, and garlic (if it agrees with you) are acceptable, but make sure butter is not used in preparation, since it adds calories and fat.
* Whereas sweet potatoes are held in high favor because of their fiber content, white potatoes, as mentioned, are unfairly maligned because of their lack of fiber. Moderate servings of white potatoes, especially in company with other vegetables, and served without butter or cream, do no harm. Baked potatoes served in restaurants (and in many homes as well) are usually of excessive size. A huge baked potato has a large amount of calories, so do not eat it. Skip the sour cream and butter served with baked potatoes. Forego or limit the salt because of its effect on hypertension (see Chapter 39). You can use chives and a bit of olive oil.
* Many restaurants serve steaks and roasts of 10, 14, or more ounces. Allow yourself to eat a lean serving of 6, 7, or 8 ounces. Take the rest home. If you are served a giant portion and want help not to eat all of it, cut the piece of steak or roast beef in half and ask for an extra plate for the portion you will take home.
* See if an appetizer on the menu can serve as your main course.
* Do not hesitate to ask for an extra plate so you can share your entree with your companion. If it is your special day when you are allowing yourself your once-per-week dessert, share your dessert, too. It is a great way to enjoy dessert while holding calories at a reasonable level.
* A national restaurant chain recently announced that it is introducing a menu with ten Weight Watchers entrees. See if one of these restaurants is near you, and patronize it. It will make it easy for you to select calorie-appropriate meals.
* In fast-food restaurants:
    1. Buy only grilled chicken sandwiches—skip the hamburgers and hot dogs.

2. Eat the grilled chicken by itself or discard the top half of the bun.
3. Forget about using ketchup—it is very high in calories.
4. Use mustard if you like—the calorie count is low.
5. Refuse french fries and all other fried products.
6. Omit huge servings of soda, which are 100 calories per eight ounces. Instead, drink water, mineral water, or, if you choose to include artificial sweeteners in your diet, have at most one 12-ounce container of artificially sweetened soda.
7. Do not even think of having a milk shake, at 450 calories each.
8. Do not even think of having ice cream desserts. They come close to milk shakes in number of calories.

Should Your Diet Include Alcohol?

This is a very important issue. It is generally agreed that alcohol in moderation may be beneficial to your heart. "Moderate" is generally considered to be four ounces of wine or one cocktail per day. It is said that red wine is the most beneficial because of a chemical in the skin of the grapes used to produce it that is not present in the production of white wine.

I have two concerns about advocating the daily consumption of alcohol. The first is addressed to everyone engaged in losing weight; the second affects us all. My first concern arises from the considerable number of calories in alcohol. Four ounces of red wine contains about 100 calories; one and one-half ounces of 80-proof liquor (the standard serving in a cocktail) contains 120 calories. A highball mix of sweet beverage will add more calories. If you plan to lose one pound per week, adding 120 alcohol calories to your food intake will require subtracting 120 additional food calories. Two drinks a day, whether wine or a cocktail, seriously hamper weight reduction. My second concern is that if you are led to believe that daily alcohol consumption is beneficial, and if you have never or only occasionally consumed alcohol before, you may wind up drinking excessively. I have seen this happen, and it is very sad. I have also known people who were already drinking who used the concept that "it is good for you" as a justification for excess drinking. It is not. Excess drinking is never good for you.

For these reasons, I do not advocate adding a moderate amount of alcohol to your diet. If you already include one glass of wine or a cocktail per day in your diet, remember its calorie count. And remember not to drink immoderately.

What about Coffee?

I disagree with the ban sometimes placed on coffee. Although some have spoken unfavorably about it from a heart standpoint for some time, many now declare it to be beneficial. I believe that if you enjoy coffee, again the rule is moderation. Drink only one or two cups a day, and do not add excess calories or fat through sugar, cream, or whole milk. Be especially aware of the coffee you choose if you are a regular patron at one of the gourmet coffee restaurants that are so popular these days. Many of the beverages offered—with large amounts of milk, whipped cream, and flavored syrups—are essentially desserts.

CHAPTER 30

How to Plan Your Own Diet

My goal in this chapter is to build on what you have learned so far and teach you (1) how to make food choices that are appropriate to your own *individual* weight-loss needs and (2) after reaching a normal weight how to make choices that will help you maintain that weight for life. Knowledge of both is essential to cholesterol control and cardiovascular risk reduction.

The Turner Weight-Loss System (see Chapter 26), the basis for the weight-loss approach I am recommending here, is not a collection of calorie-computed menus but rather a system of gradually subtracting enough high-calorie foods from what you now eat to bring about a loss of one pound per week. This means taking in 500 fewer calories per day than you expend, resulting in a subtraction of 3,500 calories per week, the amount contained in 1 pound of fat. Part of achieving this difference between intake and expenditure can readily be accomplished by increasing exercise. For example, if right now you do not exercise, using 200 calories by walking two miles per day would reduce the number of food calories you need to subtract to 300 per day instead of 500. You will find this not difficult to accomplish and maintain on a long-term basis, and it assists in cholesterol control.

When your normal weight is reached, your experience selecting food during weight loss will enable you to easily make the daily choices needed to maintain your healthy weight. And, as with weight loss, weight maintenance will be easier to sustain because, with the

Turner Weight-Loss System, instead of trying to follow a standardized menu, you will be taking your own preferences into account in making your food choices.

One of the underlying reasons so many people start and then give up on calculated diets is physiological and has to do with the way our internal appetite-control system, or appestat, works. On any given day, our appestat causes us to expect to take in an amount of food similar to the amount taken in on recent previous days. An abrupt reduction is very difficult, and people who suddenly restrict caloric intake on a calculated diet that involves severely restricting calories are likely to experience extreme—even uncontrollable—hunger.

Besides the way the appestat works, there are other reasons why calculated diets seem doomed to failure. Many calculated diets assume that there is a standardized formula with which calories can be calculated for weight loss for groups of people, based on height and gender, for example. This is unrealistic. Physical activity levels and calorie requirements vary so widely from person to person that, even for people of the same height and gender, it would be impossible to create a standardized calculated diet of exactly how many calories to consume daily. For example, it is clear that on the job, an accountant uses fewer calories per day than a carpenter.

The problem of creating a calculated diet for someone who is overweight is even more complicated because of the very fact that the person is overweight. A sizable number of calories are needed to carry excess body weight while engaging in daily activities, but to my knowledge no data exist for figuring into diet calculations how many calories are involved. Without this data, it is impossible to calculate precisely the exact number of calories required per day. Take away too many calories, and not only will the person experience extreme hunger resulting from the appestat reacting to the abrupt change, but he or she may be insufficiently nurtured to carry the excess weight.

These are among the reasons the system I am teaching is superior to the numerous fad diets you may have tried or read about. These diets are mainly based on food taken in, whereas emphasis should be on food *not* taken in. That is why I call my approach a "calorie-subtraction system." It is for the same reasons—the need to reset the appestat so calorie reduction is not so severe that people just throw in the towel and the need to be responsive to individual requirements that vary with activity level—that my system is one of *gradual* weight loss. It is a system with *moderate* calorie subtraction rather than immediately subtracting so many calories that the program is impossible to maintain long-term.

All of this is vital because of your need for a lifetime plan of weight control, including weight loss, if needed, followed by proper weight maintenance. This is why, rather than referring to what I am teaching you as a *diet,* I call it a *system of eating.* Instead of thinking of it as something with a time limit on it—which is how we generally think of diets—I want you to think of it as learning a new way of eating, a way that you will learn and commit to for life.

Planning Your Weight-Control Goals

Your first step in starting your new system of eating is to find out what your target normal weight actually should be (by *normal,* I mean the weight that is medically considered healthy). If you are of average bone structure, rather than being "big-framed" or "small-framed," the following table will provide you with the information you need:

Women: 100 pounds for the first 5 feet, with an additional 5 pounds for each additional inch of height.
Men: 106 pounds for the first 5 feet, with an additional 6 pounds for each additional inch of height.

These weights correspond very closely with those of healthy young adults who have not developed an overweight problem in their childhood or teens. People with a large bone structure will have a slightly higher-target normal weight.

Your weight-loss goal should be to reach your normal weight. I cannot condone stopping short of this; I do not agree with those professionals who say it is okay to stop several pounds short of your target normal weight. Cardiovascular disease risk begins as weight excess begins; there is no arbitrary point above "normal" when risk starts. Some people believe that it is normal to "fleshen out" as one grows older. This is not true.

Your second step is to remember that the system of eating I am teaching you for weight loss is not based on calculating and following computed calorie amounts. It is the far simpler system of *learning how to avoid food you should not eat* and removing enough calories from what you are now eating, in conjunction with increasing your exercise, in order to bring about a 500-calorie-per-day difference between calories you take in and those you expend in order to lose one pound per week.

Yes, I have said this before, but I want it to become second nature to you—so much a part of how you think that you naturally incorporate it into your life! Remember, too, that if you increase your exercise by 200 calories per day, to lose one pound per week you have to reduce your calorie intake only by 300 per day, not a difficult task. Again, the key to the calorie-subtraction system is eliminating high-calorie foods. The simplicity of the system will enable you to comfortably continue it indefinitely, until you reach your goal.

I am going to illustrate the ease and success of carrying out this system of eating by telling you about my mother. My mother was a farm woman with an eighth-grade education who baked pie or cake every day of the week, including Sunday. By the time she reached seventy, she was moderately overweight, her memory was not what it had been, and she had developed early diabetes. Her doctor advised her to lose weight. On her own initiative, despite her memory loss, she discontinued desserts, reduced her consumption of home-baked bread, reduced her food serving sizes, and reduced her breakfast bacon to one slice per day. The result: she lost all of her excess weight, her diabetes went away, and she lived a more healthy life well into her eighties.

Selecting Your Own Foods for Weight Loss

After having emphasized so strongly that this is not a diet manual with calculated diets, I need to explain why I am including two diet menus in this chapter. They were adapted from my early Cardiac No. 1 (1,200-calorie) and my Cardiac No. 2 (1,800-calorie) diets that proved so unsuccessful when prescribed.

When I painfully observed the failure of my hard work with the calculated diets, I switched my patients to the plan that was proving successful in my own weight-reduction effort: simply avoiding obviously high-calorie foods. This successful experience is what enabled me to deduce that both the 1,200-calorie and the 1,800-calorie diets were too low for continuing weight-reduction compliance, and that the wide variation in the calorie expenditure of my patients made the use of any one standard diet impossible; in other words, "one size did not fit all."

However, I found the 1,200- and 1,800-calorie diet menus proved valuable when used in a different way—not as models people should copy food by food and amount by amount but as examples they could use when creating their own meals because they showed patients what a balanced diet really is, they showed the omission of high-calorie foods, and they showed moderation.

Do not try to live by these menus; rather, use them for inspiration and general guidance. I have included midmorning and midafternoon snacks in these menus not because I necessarily recommend snacking but because many people would abandon a diet without snack suggestions. If snacks are not part of your daily eating habits, there is no reason to start snacking now unless it will help you subtract calories at mealtimes, since snacks add calories unless you use no-calorie items.

To assist my patients in choosing high-calorie foods to eliminate, I provided them with a calorie chart listing foods with the corresponding number of calories. An expanded version of this chart, which also lists protein, carbohydrate, and fat contents of foods, is included following the sample 1,200- and 1,800-calorie diet menus.

As you will see, numerous high-calorie foods can be eliminated without severely disrupting your meals. Again, these include high-calorie desserts, especially pie, cake, and ice cream; fried foods of all kinds; more than one or two slices of bread daily and the accompanying butter; fat that can be removed from meat, chicken, and turkey; sugar- or fructose-sweetened soft drinks; oversized hamburgers, especially those prepared with meat of high fat content; hot dogs and luncheon meats; and high-calorie sauces and salad dressings. Notwithstanding the nutrient value of olive oil and macadamia-nut oil, they are high in calories and should be used in very limited amounts.

As you gradually reduce your intake of high-calorie foods, you will be pleased to find your appetite for them steadily diminishing, making it progressively easy to abstain from them. This change is the result of resetting your appestat at a lower level. When you eliminate high-calorie sweets—which are high in carbohydrates—it also results in breaking the vicious cycle of hypoglycemia. This means that even though at first you will miss the high-calorie foods you eliminate, it will not take long before not eating these foods feels natural and you no longer crave them. This is physiological as well as psychological: you are actually resetting your body's appestat and changing your metabolic pattern as well as getting used to new eating habits. In my own case, my craving for apple pie once or twice daily soon ceased. Now I am quite happy with one moderate dessert a week.

Your Current Diet

What if your current diet includes many high-calorie and high-cholesterol foods? This is a very important question—a question that applies to many of us. To answer it, I will use the example of one of my patients. After we discussed his commitment to lose weight by expending 500 calories per day more than he took in, he told me his daily diet included not one high-calorie food but several, and many of them were high in cholesterol, too. "I eat pancakes, french toast, or a big sweet roll for breakfast, hamburger on a bun with french fries and a milk shake at lunch, fried chicken or steak with a lot of fat at dinner, and I have pie or cake twice a day," he told me. "Am I supposed to just cut out 300 calories per day and increase my exercise by 200 calories? What about all the other high-calorie foods? And what about all the foods that are high in cholesterol?"

My answer to this crucial question is based on everything that you have read so far. Your first step is to eliminate one high-calorie food per day, amounting to 300 calories, while expending 200 additional calories through increased exercise. *This* is the commitment you must make to lose one pound per week—and that is your goal. Subtracting more calories makes weight loss not easier but more difficult. As I have explained, suddenly eliminating a large number of calories will cause you to experience extreme hunger, which makes you more likely to throw in the towel. I want to guide you to a weight loss system that you can sustain and therefore be successful with. This means you must focus primarily on week-to-week and month-to-month goals, and recognize that getting rid of an appreciable amount of excess weight may well take several months or even a year or two, and that during that time your risk of a heart attack and stroke will steadily decrease.

So if you are subtracting only one high-calorie food per day from your current diet, what do you do about those other high-calorie foods that are so often high in cholesterol, too? The answer is that you bear in mind everything you have learned so far, commit to reducing the cholesterol in your diet, and, at your own pace, substitute healthier alternatives for high-cholesterol foods. And you do this on your own schedule. Just as you are gradually losing weight, you *gradually* change your food choices to the healthy choices you now know about.

Maintaining Your Weight

When you have reached your goal, how do you maintain your weight? The answer to this question is simple: by the time you have achieved your target normal weight, you will have become very experienced knowing what foods to avoid or diminish, using the charts I am providing for reference. This knowledge will enable you to add back in limited amounts some of the healthy foods you have been omitting in order to subtract calories for weight loss. This will require some practice, but you can do it.

If you eat too much one week and regain weight you have lost, you can eat less the next. There will be variations in food needs and food intake resulting from changes in physical activity or workload, periods of increased personal stress, and a variable frequency of social activities involving food, all of which you can deal with in the same manner: if you eat more one day, or one week, you will eat less the next day or week. As I have observed during my own long experience with this system of eating, well-deserved indulgences during vacations can easily be offset upon returning home.

If you commit to the system of calorie subtraction, gradual weight loss, and weight maintenance I am recommending, combined with gradually replacing unhealthy foods with healthy foods, you will have changed your eating habits for life, and maintaining them will be natural for you. Keep in mind that making this extremely important commitment may save your life or reduce disability from a heart attack or stroke.

In medical practice, I have experienced great pleasure in seeing hundreds of men and women achieve their targeted weight loss and maintain a healthy, normal weight. Some of these people were returning to their trim appearance of early life, and others were slender for the first time. All of them felt better about themselves for making the commitment to health, for having a more attractive appearance, for being able to enjoy physical activities without the strain that excess weight creates, and for having a far broader range of fashions to wear. I have experienced the same positive results in my own weight loss and maintenance. I wish you success in your venture to change your eating habits for life!

Table 30.1.
Sample 1200-calorie and 1800-calorie menus

✷ Sample 1200-Calorie Menu

40% Carbohydrate
30% Protein
30% Fat

Breakfast

- Fresh fruit	0.5 cup
- Milk, skim, with added vitamins A and D	1 cup
- Egg whites	2 or 3
- Precut breakfast steaks or other lean meat such as cured ham, extra lean, 4% fat, or Canadian bacon	2 ounces
- Oil, olive or macadamia	1 tsp.

Morning Snack

- Nuts, raw almonds, unsalted	2 Tbsp.
or	
- Whole-grain bread or toast	1 slice
(with nonhydrogenated margarine or olive or macadamia oil if not part of breakfast)	1 tsp.

Lunch

- Chicken breast fillet, grilled	3 ounces
- Salad, mixed greens, raw	2 cups
- Salad dressing (1 Tbsp. olive or macadamia-nut oil and lemon juice or apple cider vinegar)	
- Yogurt, nonfat	8 ounces
- Fresh fruit (apple, pear, peach)	1

Afternoon Snack

- Celery stalk, small, 5 inches long, raw	2 each

Dinner

- Fish, salmon, Atlantic, fillet, baked or broiled, or lean beef, chicken, turkey, or pork	3 ounces
- Broccoli, spear, 5 inches long, cooked	2 each
- Salad, mixed greens, raw	1 cup
- Salad dressing (1 Tbsp. olive or macadamia-nut oil and lemon juice or apple cider vinegar)	
- Crackers, wheat, garden herb, organic, low-fat	5 each
- Yogurt, nonfat, or low-fat cottage cheese	0.5 cup
- Blueberries, fresh	1 cup

✷ Sample 1,800-Calorie Menu

40% Carbohydrate
30% Protein
30% Fat

Breakfast

- Whole fruit, fresh	0.5 cup
- Milk, skim, with added vitamins A and D	1 cup
- Egg whites	2 or 3
- Precut breakfast steaks or other lean meat such as cured ham, extra lean, 4% fat, or Canadian bacon	4 ounces
- Bread or toast, whole-wheat or other whole grain	1 slice
- Oil, olive or macadamia	1 tsp.
- Cheese, mozzarella, low-moisture, 50% less fat	0.5 ounce

Morning Snack

- Nuts, raw almonds, unsalted	3 Tbsp.
or	
- Whole-grain bread or toast	1 slice
(with nonhydrogenated margarine or olive or macadamia oil if not part of breakfast)	1 tsp.

Lunch

- Chicken breast fillet, grilled	3 ounces

- Salad, mixed greens, raw	2 cups
- Salad dressing (2 Tbsp. olive or macadamia-nut oil and lemon juice or apple cider vinegar)	
- Crackers, wheat, garden herb, organic, low-fat	4-6
- Yogurt, nonfat	8 ounces
- Fresh fruit (apple, pear, peach)	1

Afternoon Snack

- Carrots, baby, raw	0.25 cup
- Celery, stalk, small, 5 inches long, raw	3 each
- Cheese, string, mozzarella, sticks, reduced-fat, low-moisture	1 each

Dinner

- Fish, salmon, Atlantic, fillet, baked or broiled, or lean beef, pork, chicken, or turkey	5 ounces
- Broccoli, spear, 5 inches long, cooked	3 each
- Salad, mixed greens, raw	1 cup
- Salad dressing (2 Tbsp. olive or macadamia-nut oil and lemon juice or apple cider vinegar)	
- Whole-grain brown and wild seasoned blend, dry	1 serving
- Yogurt, nonfat, or low-fat cottage cheese	0.5 cup
- Blueberries, fresh	1 cup

Table 30.2.
Calorie chart (including protein, carbohydrate, and fat contents per gram)

Reading and keeping on hand the chart below will help you to make choices about high-calorie foods to eliminate from your diet and familiarize yourself with the protein, carbohydrate, and fat contents of foods in order to approximate the 30/40/30 formula for a heart and blood-vessel healthy diet.

Source: USDA National Nutrient Database for Standard Reference, Release 18 (2005) http://www.ars.usda.gov/nutrientdata.

Food Item	Amount	Calories	Carbs grams	Protein grams	Fat grams
Fruit					
Apple, raw, with skin	1 large	110	29.28	0.55	0.36
Applesauce, canned, unsweetened	1 cup	105	27.55	0.41	0.12
Blueberries, raw, unsweetened	1 cup	83	21.01	1.07	0.48
Cantaloupe, raw	1 cup balls	60	14.44	1.49	0.34
Grapefruit, pink	one half	52	13.11	0.95	0.17
Grapes	1 cup	110	28.96	1.15	0.26
Mango	1 medium	135	35.19	1.06	0.56
Nectarine, raw	1 2–1/2 in	60	14.35	1.44	0.44
Orange, raw	1 large	86	21.62	1.73	0.22
Peaches, raw	1 large	61	14.98	1.43	0.39
Pear, raw	1 medium	96	25.66	0.63	0.2
Pineapple, raw	1 cup	74	19.58	0.84	0.19

Food Item	Amount	Calories	Carbs grams	Protein grams	Fat grams
Pineapple, chunks, canned, juice pack, drained	1 cup	109	28.16	0.92	0.2
Raspberries, raw	1 cup	64	14.69	1.48	0.8
Strawberries, raw, whole	1 cup	46	11.06	0.96	0.43
Watermelon, raw	1 cup balls	46	11.63	0.94	0.23
Grains					
Bread, white	1 slice	66	12.65	1.91	0.82
Bread, whole wheat	1 slice	69	12.91	2.72	1.18
Biscuits	1 2-1/2"	212	26.76	4.2	9.76
Cereal, oats, cooked	1 cup	147	25.27	6.08	2.34
Cereal, ready-to-eat, rice	1 cup	56	12.57	0.88	0.07
Cereal, ready-to-eat, wheat flakes	1 cup	106	24.30	3	0.96
Cereal, ready-to-eat, wheat, shredded	1 cup	167	40.67	5.05	0.54
Crackers, snack-type, square	5	100	12.20	1.5	5.05
English muffin	1	140	27.38	5.37	1.05
Rice, white, cooked	1/2 cup	103	22.25	2.12	0.22
Rice, brown, cooked	1/2 cup	108	22.33	2.5	0.88
Granola bar, plain	1 bar	118	16.10	2.54	4.95

Food Item	Amount	Calories	Carbs grams	Protein grams	Fat grams
Meat, Fish, Poultry					
Beef, top sirloin, broiled	3 oz	170	0.00	29.34	4.96
Beef, tenderloin, select, broiled	3 oz	194	0.00	29.07	7.76
Beef, top round, lean, braised	3 oz	199	0.00	36.12	5
Beef, chuck, arm roast, lean, braised	3 oz	195	0.00	33.37	5.8
Beef, ground 95% lean, pan-broiled	3 oz	164	0.00	25.8	5.94
Beef, ground 90% lean, pan-broiled	3 oz	204	0.00	25.21	10.68
Beef, ground, 85% lean, pan-broiled	3 oz	232	0.00	24.62	14.02
Beef, ground, 80% lean, pan-broiled	3 oz	246	0.00	24.04	15.94
Beef, ground, 75% lean, pan-broiled	3 oz	248	0.00	23.45	16.44
Beef, liver, cooked, pan-fried	3 oz	175	5.16	26.52	4.68
Chicken breast, oven-roasted, fat-free, sliced	3 oz	79	2.17	16.79	0.39
Chicken breast, meat only, roasted	3 oz	165	0.00	31.02	3.57
Chicken thigh, meat only, roasted	3 oz	209	0.00	25.94	10.88

Food Item	Amount	Calories	Carbs grams	Protein grams	Fat grams
Turkey, light meat, roasted	3 oz	157	0.00	29.9	3.22
Turkey ham, extra lean, deli	3 oz	118	1.50	19.6	3.8
Ham, cured extra lean (5% fat), roasted	3 oz	145	1.50	20.93	5.53
Ham, cured regular (11% fat), roasted	3 oz	178	0.00	22.62	9.02
Pork, loin, lean only, roasted	3 oz	240	0.00	28.71	13.06
Pork, shoulder, lean only, roasted	3 oz	230	0.00	25.33	13.54
Lamb, trimmed to 1/8-inch fat, cooked	3 oz	271	0.00	25.51	18.01
Salmon, Atlantic, wild, cooked, dry heat	3 oz	182	0.00	25.44	8.13
Salmon, Atlantic, farmed, cooked, dry heat	3 oz	206	0.00	22.1	12.35
Salmon, pink, canned, drained solids with bone	3 oz	136	0.00	23.08	4.83
Tuna, fresh, cooked, dry heat	3 oz	139	0.00	29.97	1.22
Tuna, light, canned in water, drained	3 oz	116	0.00	25.51	0.82
Fish, roughy, orange, cooked, dry heat	3 oz	105	0.00	22.64	0.9

Food Item	Amount	Calories	Carbs grams	Protein grams	Fat grams
Fish, cod, Atlantic, cooked, dry heat	3 oz	105	0.00	22.83	0.86
Fish, flounder and sole, cooked, dry heat	3 oz	117	0.00	24.16	1.53
Fish, catfish, farmed, cooked, dry heat	3 oz	152	0.00	18.72	8.02
Fish, catfish, wild, cooked, dry heat	3 oz	105	0.00	18.47	2.85
Shrimp, cooked, moist heat	3 oz	99	0.00	20.91	1.08
Shrimp, imitation, made from surimi	3 oz	101	0.00	12.39	1.47
Lobster, cooked, moist heat	3 oz	98	1.28	20.5	0.59
Egg, whole, large (50 grams)	1 large	74	0.38	6.26	4.95
Milk, Cheese, Yogurt, Ice Cream					
Milk, nonfat, fluid	1 cup	83	12.15	8.26	0.2
Milk, low-fat, fluid, 1% milkfat	1 cup	102	12.18	8.22	2.37
Milk, reduced fat, fluid, 2% milkfat	1 cup	122	11.42	8.05	4.81
Milk, whole, 3.25% milkfat	1 cup	146	11.03	7.86	7.93
Soy milk, fluid	1 cup	127	12.08	10.98	4.7

Food Item	Amount	Calories	Carbs grams	Protein grams	Fat grams
Cheese, American	1 oz	110			9
Cheese, cottage, low-fat, 1% milkfat	1 cup	163	6.15	28	2.31
Cheese, cottage, low-fat 2% milkfat	1 cup	203	8.20	31.05	4.36
Cheese, mozzarella, part skim	1 oz	72	0.79	6.88	4.51
Cheese, ricotta, part skim	1/2 cup	171	6.37	14.12	9.81
Yogurt, plain, skim milk	1 cup	137	18.82	14.04	0.44
Ice cream, vanilla	1/2 cup	145	16.99	2.52	7.92
Ice cream, light	1/2 cup	105	14.57	2.7	5.07
Nuts					
Nuts, almonds, dry roasted	1/4 cup	206	6.65	7.62	18.23
Nuts, pecans, dry roasted	1/4 cup	171	3.43	2.27	17.8
Nuts, walnuts, English	1/4 cup	163	3.43	3.81	16.3
Peanuts, dry roasted	1/4 cup	214	7.85	8.64	18.13
Peanut butter	2 Tbsp.	188	6.26	8.03	16.12

Food Item	Amount	Calories	Carbs grams	Protein grams	Fat grams
Oils and Fats					
Butter	1 Tbsp.	102	0.01	0.12	11.52
Margarine	1 Tbsp.	104	0.12	0.12	11.34
Oil, olive	1 Tbsp.	119	0.00	0	13.5
Oil, canola	1 Tbsp.	124	0.00	0	14
Pies, cakes, cookies					
Cake, angel food	1 piece	72	16.18	1.65	0.22
Cake, chocolate	1 piece	235	34.94	2.62	10.5
Cake, yellow	1 piece	239	37.63	2.24	9.28
Cookies, chocolate chip	1 cookie	59	8.18	0.59	2.71
Cookies, brownies	1 square	227	35.78	2.69	9.13
Pie, apple	1 slice (1/6)	277	39.78	2.22	12.87
Vegetables					
Beans, green, canned, drained	1 cup	27	6.08	1.55	0.14
Broccoli, flower clusters, raw	1 cup	20	3.72	2.12	0.25
Broccoli, frozen, chopped, cooked	1 cup	52	9.84	5.7	0.22
Cabbage, raw, shredded	1 cup	17	3.91	1.01	0.08

Food Item	Amount	Calories	Carbs grams	Protein grams	Fat grams
Cabbage, cooked, drained	1 cup	16	3.35	0.77	0.32
Carrots, raw	1 cup	50	11.69	1.13	0.29
Cauliflower, raw	1 cup	25	5.30	1.98	0.1
Cauliflower, cooked, boiled, drained	1 cup	12	2.22	0.99	0.24
Corn, sweet canned, whole kernel	1 cup	133	30.49	4.3	1.64
Lettuce, iceberg	1 cup	8	1.63	0.49	0.08
Lettuce, Romaine	1 cup	8	1.54	0.58	0.14
Lettuce, leaf	1 cup	5	1.00	0.49	0.05
Peas, green, frozen, cooked	1 cup	62	11.41	4.12	0.22
Peas, edible-podded, boiled	1 cup	67	11.28	5.23	0.37
Peppers, sweet, green, raw, sliced	1 cup	18	4.27	0.79	0.16
Potatoes, baked, flesh	1 medium	145	33.62	3.06	0.16
Pumpkin, canned	1 cup	83	19.82	2.69	1.37
Spinach, raw	1 cup	7	1.09	0.86	0.12
Spinach, frozen, chopped, cooked	1/2 cup	30	4.90	3.81	0.47

Food Item	Amount	Calories	Carbs grams	Protein grams	Fat grams
Squash, winter, spaghetti, cooked	1 cup	42	10.01	1.02	0.4
Squash, winter, butternut, baked	1 cup	82	21.50	1.84	0.18
Squash, winter, acorn, baked	1 cup	115	29.89	2.3	0.29
Squash, summer, cooked	1 cup	36	7.76	1.64	0.56
Squash, summer, raw, sliced	1 cup	18	3.79	1.37	0.2
Sweet potato, baked	1 medium	103	23.61	2.29	0.17
Tomatoes, raw, sliced	1 cup	32	5.84	1.58	0.36
Tomatoes, canned, whole	1/2 cup	23	5.24	1.1	0.16
Dried Beans and Lentils					
Beans, great northern, canned	1 cup	299	55.10	19.31	1.02
Beans, kidney, canned	1 cup	218	39.91	13.44	0.87
Beans, navy, canned	1 cup	296	53.58	19.73	1.13
Chickpeas (garbanzo beans), canned	1 cup	286	54.29	11.88	2.74
Lentils, mature seeds, cooked	1 cup	14	2.48	1.11	0.05

Food Item	Amount	Calories	Carbs grams	Protein grams	Fat grams
Beverages					
Beer, lite	12 fl oz	103	5.81	0.85	0
Beer, regular	12 fl oz	153	12.64	1.64	0
Soda, regular	12 fl oz	136	35.18	0.26	0.07
Soda, diet	12 fl oz	7	0.11	0.39	0.11
Wine	5 fl oz	124	4.03	0.1	0

Familiarizing Yourself with Cholesterol Content

The following chart contains the cholesterol content of certain key foods and will also be of use to you in creating your heart and blood-vessel healthy diet. In reviewing the amount of cholesterol these foods contain, remember that the AHA recommends an ideal cholesterol intake of 200 mgs. and an upper limit of 300 mgs. of cholesterol per day. See which foods you would include in a typical day's meals to reach the ideal or maximum amount.

Cholesterol Content of Meat, Fish, and Poultry	
Food Item **per 100 grams (3 oz)**	**Cholesterol** **mg**
Beef, top sirloin, broiled	46
Beef, tenderloin, select, broiled	73
Beef, top round, lean, braised	90
Beef, chuck, arm roast, lean, braised	57
Beef, ground 95% lean, pan-broiled	76
Beef, ground 90% lean, pan-broiled	82
Beef, ground, 85% lean, pan-broiled	86
Beef, ground, 80% lean, pan-broiled	90
Beef, ground, 75% lean, pan-broiled	93
Beef, ground, 70% lean, pan-broiled	95
Beef, liver, cooked, pan-fried	381
Chicken breast, oven-roasted, fat-free, sliced	36
Chicken breast, meat only, roasted	85
Chicken thigh, meat only, roasted	95
Turkey, light meat, roasted	69
Turkey ham, extra lean, deli	67
Ham, cured extra lean (5% fat), roasted	53
Ham, cured regular (11% fat), roasted	59
Pork, loin, lean only, roasted	81
Pork, shoulder, lean only, roasted	90
Lamb, trimmed to 1/8-inch fat, cooked	96
Salmon, Atlantic, wild, cooked, dry heat	71
Salmon, Atlantic, farmed, cooked, dry heat	63

Food Item per 100 grams (3 oz)	**Cholesterol mg**
Salmon, pink, canned, drained solids with bone	82
Tuna, fresh, cooked, dry heat	58
Tuna, light, canned in water, drained	30
Fish, roughy, orange, cooked, dry heat	80
Fish, cod, Atlantic, cooked, dry heat	55
Fish, flounder and sole, cooked, dry heat	68
Fish, catfish, farmed, cooked, dry heat	64
Fish, catfish, wild, cooked, dry heat	72
Shrimp, cooked, moist heat	195
Shrimp, imitation, made from surimi	36
Lobster, cooked, moist heat	72
Egg, whole, large (50 grams)	211

Source: USDA National Nutrient Database for Standard Reference, Release 18 (2005) http://www.ars.usda.gov/nutrientdata.

Note: I want to thank two people who have helped so much in bringing this crucial chapter together: First, Frances, my wife of more than fifty years, who received a degree in home economics from what is now Missouri State University. She has kept me continuously on a balanced diet, always explaining how and why she is making specific food choices. This gave me expert professional guidance in dealing with my patients throughout my career and has extended into writing this chapter.

I would also like to thank Helen C. Reid, Ph.D., RD/LD, associate dean and professor, College of Health and Human Services, Missouri State University, Springfield. Reid researched extensively to enable us to jointly prepare the 1,200- and 1,800-calorie sample diet menus to demonstrate the balance and proportions of foods from different categories. She worked with me to integrate features of my previous diets with hers and came up with the food ratio percentages recommended by Krauss. She also provided the expanded chart showing the content of calories, protein, carbohydrate, and fat of many foods and the chart "Cholesterol Content of Meat, Fish, and Poultry."

CHAPTER 31

Support Groups versus Food-Based Programs

For most of us, checking in regularly with someone and reporting on our weight-loss process is a great help in maintaining our commitment. This is why, in addition to his or her medical expertise, I have recommended involving your personal physician in your weight-loss process as much as your health plan permits. If you find your plan does not allow physician appointments for weight loss, check to see if it will cover doctor appointments for a cholesterol-lowering diet, which may be covered under a different category.

Of course, allying yourself on a long-term basis with your personal physician involves more than just weight control. Your other needs include blood pressure control (see Chapter 39); blood lipid assay and, if abnormal, correction (see Chapters 36 and 37); and attention to the other risks you are learning about in this book.

I have mentioned that I have advised some of my patients with weight-loss goals to supplement their visits to me by joining a weight-loss organization for the support it offers. If you need to lose weight, you may benefit from joining such a group. Weight Watchers is the most well known of these. Currently, there are twenty thousand Weight Watchers meetings in the United States per year. Weight loss is the goal, and meetings entail weight-loss instruction and support. Although cholesterol control is not focused on specifically, their "food points" suggestions are declared to be heart healthy.

It is important for you to know that if you join Weight Watchers, you will be required to follow its suggested food-points plan. Since they are health oriented and not extreme in their calorie reduction, if you find the support of meetings valuable, following the plan is fine.

Weight Watchers advises that weight loss does not exceed two pounds per week. As you know, I recommend that for most people a reasonable goal is one pound per week. A two-pound-per-week goal may be desirable for people who are severely overweight. The reason I have not emphasized this is that some severely overweight people are more successful with the more moderate goal of one pound per week—and I do not want people to feel that they are failing, because they are not failing; they may simply have set too high a goal. At the same time, if you join Weight Watchers and find its plan easy to follow, the goal of two pounds per week may be feasible and, from a medical point of view, is not unhealthy.

Other support organizations include Overeaters Anonymous, which has sixty-five hundred meeting groups in more than fifty countries, and TOPS, with ten thousand chapters worldwide.

If you join a weight-loss organization for regular check-ins and support, the frequency of your doctor visits must not be reduced.

I do not recommend "food-based" or "meal-replacement" weight-loss programs, where prepackaged foods are sold to weight-loss customers. In my experience, these programs have not shown as good results long-term as those of weight-loss organizations such as Weight Watchers.

Some food-based programs offer periodic group discussion sessions, but I question the effectiveness of them, conducted in a sales-setting environment. Also, the transition from prepackaged food to regular food frequently fails, with customers regaining the weight they lost, often becoming heavier than before because of overeating, despite their lowered appestats, after returning to food that is so much more enjoyable to them. These programs cannot be followed long-term. This is why I recommend the more gradual approach of lowering your daily intake of calories with the kind of system my patients and I used.

Remember: In weight control, the crucial thing is not to lose many pounds quickly, but rather to lose pounds and keep them off so that you can reach and maintain your desired weight. Although quick weight loss may be temporarily impressive, slow but consistent weight loss usually accomplishes the goal.

CHAPTER 32

More Tips for Dieting

Here is a summary of the additional advice for dieting that I shared with my patients: First, buy an accurate scale with readings down to at least one-half pound and markers that are clearly visible to you with your present level of visual acuity. If you are embarking on a program to lose weight, I urge you to consider purchasing a scale of the quality used in your physician's office. These scales come in two types: balance (with an eye-level horizontal beam, graduated in quarter pounds) and digital (with a waist-level, large-size electronic screen to display weights clearly). These scales are expensive but will give you a lifetime of valuable service. (An excellent brand is DETECTO. Pricing information is available through Bach Medical Supply, 417–883-1400.) A less expensive alternative is the digital scale endorsed by Weight Watchers. This scale is accurate to .2 pounds and shows your weight on a wireless detachable screen so you can read it easily. The more commonly used lower-priced floor-based scales have a spring-operated mechanism that is subject to humidity and temperature changes, and their accuracy is uncertain. Even if they have large dials, often it is difficult, if not impossible, to tell within a pound or two whether you have gained or lost. This prevents accurate measurement of weight, and it deprives you of the much deserved pride of recognizing that you have lost even half a pound.

Second, weigh yourself once weekly on the same day every week, before breakfast, unclothed, ideally after urinating and having a bowel movement. Weighing more often and at other hours may reveal daily body-fluid fluctuations that will add to your weight, and this may cause unnecessary stress. Variations in body-fluid content, especially in women before menstrual periods, occur naturally.

Third, treasure even a half pound of weight loss. Do not lose heart when you gain a pound or fail to lose.

Fourth, keep a tape measure in the bathroom and check your abdominal circumference at the level of your navel after you weigh. The measurement will be less at this hour than at any later time of the day. Because of the high risk attributed to excess abdominal fat, it is extremely important that men reduce their abdominal circumference to below forty inches and that women reduce theirs to below thirty-five inches. Write down your weight and abdominal measurement on a card and take it with you on visits with your physician.

Fifth, establish short-term goals: week to week and month to month. Physician-supervised programs work best with initial visits no more than four to six weeks apart (and rarely succeed if visits are more than six to eight weeks apart).

Sixth, allow yourself a special meal once a week, with dessert if desired (but not pie à la mode or other desserts that are actually two desserts masquerading as one!).

Seventh, allow some weight gain on vacations—a two- or three-pound increase can soon be eliminated.

Eighth, if you do not show desired progress in two to four months, consider joining Weight Watchers, TOPS, Overeaters Anonymous, or another reputable weight-loss organization that will provide you with regular support meetings.

Ninth, learn to appreciate your achievement in losing pound by pound even though your goal may seem far away.

Tenth, should you fail to lose or if you lose less than your goal amount between one meeting with your doctor and the next, do not break your appointment with your doctor. He or she will be respectful and helpful—we are all human.

Eleventh, concerning your choice of weight-loss plans, remember that your success depends on your consistently maintaining a calorie intake that is less than your calorie expenditure, and that the difference must amount to 500 calories per day if you are to lose a pound a week.

And finally, remember that few people succeed in losing weight without a regular exercise regime. Adopting an exercise program such as the one I suggest in the next chapter will help you strike a balance between cutting calories and using up more calories through increasing physical activity.

CHAPTER 33

What Is a Proper Exercise Program?

We all need exercise. It improves heart and lung efficiency, maintains healthy cholesterol and triglyceride levels or reduces them if they are too high, controls body weight and blood pressure, and manages diabetes. Because exercise is so crucial for all of us, one of my major concerns is that today the great majority of us do not exercise adequately. Perhaps there is too much contradictory information floating around; people are not sure exactly what to do, and they use their lack of answers as an excuse to do nothing. How much exercise is best? What kind should it be? What equipment should be used? The tremendous attention given to exercise in the media and the seemingly endless choices may be intimidating and put people off. The purpose of this chapter is to clear the air and help you to make simple, practical choices about how you can exercise effectively and make it a regular part of your life. Keep this in mind: *The combination of weight loss and increased exercise is the solution to metabolic syndrome because together they considerably reduce these risk factors for atherosclerotic diseases.*

I am going to address this chapter primarily to those of you—and remember, statistics say it is the majority—who exercise insufficiently or not at all. But first I want to clarify a point about exercise that I made in the previous chapter. I stated that it is best to go on a weight-loss plan while simultaneously increasing your exercise level. As I have explained, besides benefiting cardiovascular health, increased exercise results in a greater expenditure of calories, which, combined with reducing your calorie intake, results in weight loss. If you are overweight and you are already exercising at or above the level I am recommending here, you have to further increase your exercise level in order to lose weight. This will mean increasing the time you spend exercising.

Exercise Does Not Have to Be Difficult to Be Effective

Some fitness advocates give complex formulas to calculate the proper heart rate during exercise. They advise that if you do not exercise to nearly full capacity for sustained periods, you will not achieve any cardiovascular benefit. They usually advise doubling your resting heart rate and frequently prescribe jogging or running for extended periods at speeds greater than four miles per hour to accomplish this. I disagree with this practice. *Exercise at any level is beneficial, and, contrary to popular belief, you do not have to do it all during one session—it is the total for the day that counts.* A recent study of thousands of women showed that moderate exercise, such as walking at the comfortable rate of two miles per hour, conveys worthwhile cardiac benefits, disputing the claim that more vigorous activity is necessary.[1] Comparable studies of men have not been reported, but there is no reason to believe that men respond differently.

An onslaught of advertising has given many people the impression that adequate exercise programs require enrollment in expensive fitness centers with costly equipment. This is another misconception. Home routines are effective. Few patrons of fitness centers sustain their initial commitment to exercise there for more than several weeks or a few months. If you want to join a gym, YMCAs and YWCAs offer individual and family memberships and provide a broad range of physical activity. Reduced rates are available for those with a small income. Most YMCAs and YWCAs provide swimming, tennis, gymnasiums for sports, walking and running tracks, and a variety of exercise equipment. If you are interested in any of these activities, you can research the calories you will expend doing them.

My recommendation is that instead of calculating and attempting to reach a set high-heart-rate goal—which involves vigorous, prolonged exercise that many of you would consider work, and would therefore postpone (perhaps indefinitely)—you should set a more modest, yet still beneficial, goal. The physical activity you choose should be pleasant, available daily, and not so fatiguing that it makes you severely limit the duration.

As I have mentioned, in my experience, and as studies confirm, for most people with or without heart disease the answer is simple and inexpensive: WALKING. You can work up from slow walking for short distances to longer-distance brisk walking. If you have a heart or lung problem, your doctor can advise the proper amount and pace. For most people, the ideal is to build up to two to four miles per hour and to walk two to four miles per day six or seven days per week. As long as you follow this prescription for walking at least four days per week, you will still achieve a benefit. Walking at this rate over this distance utilizes considerable calories and is beneficial to the circulation.

If not specified by your doctor, you can tell what speed and distance works for you by heeding the natural signs of overexertion: shortness of breath and fatigue. If your speed tires you, slow down and walk for a shorter distance. You may be able to increase both speed and distance gradually over a period of time.

Walking outdoors is refreshing if the weather permits and the area is safe. You can vary your routes for changes of scenery, measuring the distances you walk either before or after by using your car odometer. Indoor walking areas in gyms are sometimes available, but many people find them monotonous.

Inclement weather, work schedules that make outdoor walking impractical, and limited time for exercise have generated a thriving market for excellent treadmills. These machines provide a handy walking surface in the home, usable at any hour for whatever time is available. I have used treadmills since their introduction at an AHA meeting almost four decades ago, and they have made it easy for me to exercise, regardless of weather and time schedule.

If you decide to purchase one, a two-horsepower motor-driven treadmill with speeds from zero to ten miles per hour costs around three hundred dollars. Do not buy a model that is *not* motor driven. Keep the walking surface of your treadmill level. If your model has a built-in upgrade elevation, block up the low end so that you are walking on a level surface. (Walking uphill requires more effort, and you would not be able to walk as long.) Dial the speed to your comfort, ideally two to four miles per hour. Heart-rate meters come with some treadmills. Use them if you like, but they are not essential.

You may walk a few minutes or up to a half hour or an hour at a time. Remember, the day's total is what matters. I am going to say this again because it is so important: *the day's total exercise is what matters.* You do not have to walk a half hour, for example, in one session; if it is more convenient, you can do it in three ten-minute increments.

Do not exercise sooner than one hour after any meal. More heart problems occur in the few hours after waking, apparently because the nervous system is adjusting from sleep to daytime activity. Some physicians advise deferring significant exercise, except as required by work, until midmorning or later, especially if early exercise brings on chest discomfort. With a treadmill, many people find it convenient to get in six or seven sessions of exercise per week. An added value: a treadmill exercise session can provide you with an opportunity to watch videos or television or listen to music.

Although most health-insurance policies do not cover the purchase of a treadmill, with a doctor's prescription you may be able to declare the medical expense as a tax deduction. Check with your accountant.

Remember that a long-term weight-control program rarely succeeds without a year-round exercise program, and for you to commit to a year-round exercise program the exercise must be pleasant for you. As support for my recommendation of walking to those of you who do not currently exercise adequately, I am going to remind you of the weight-loss formula I provided earlier that combines cutting calories from food intake with expending calories by walking.

Walking one mile uses about 100 calories. The ideal rate of weight loss is one pound per week (except for obese people and those who *choose* to commit to subtracting more calories per week to lose weight faster; remember, it is a *choice,* not a necessity, to lose more than one pound per week). One pound of body fat contains 3,500 calories. This weight loss is accomplished by reducing daily calorie-intake below calories expended by 500 calories.

You can adjust the amount of walking you do on a particular day to offset inescapable variations in eating and days of missed exercise. In other words, you can walk more to walk off additional calories that you have taken in from a larger-than-normal meal, and you can also walk more to make up for a prior day when you may have not been able to exercise. As mentioned, the ideal is to exercise daily, preferably not fewer than six days per week and never fewer than four.

7 days
x 500 calories less per day in diet
3,500 calories less per week in diet = 1 pound

If you increase the calories you expend per day by 250 by walking two and a half miles, you have to reduce daily food calories by only 250 to reach your goal of 3,500 calories less per week. This goal is easy to attain and to sustain.

7 days
x 250 calories per day used in walking two and a half miles
1,750 calories per week used in walking

7 days
X *250 calories less per day*
1,750 calories less per week in diet

1,750 calories per week used in walking
+ 1,750 calories less per week in diet
3,500 calories less per week = 1 pound

Do not overlook the importance of finding opportunities to increase physical exercise as you go about your day's activities. Walking and using stairs more often as you go about your day help more than you may realize. Bicycling instead of driving may be an appealing way to add additional exercise.

What about "Total-Body Strengthening"?

You may have heard about "total-body strengthening" and the equipment to accomplish it. Most of our ease of functioning and our endurance depend on strength in the lower part of the body. This is best enhanced by walking. Muscle building in the upper body produces fewer benefits unless your job or your hobbies require much use of the arm and shoulder muscles.

Some fitness writers advocate weight lifting for cardiovascular benefit. Lifting is chiefly *isometric* exercise (muscle tightening with limited movement), which raises the blood pressure and should be avoided except under professional supervision. *Aerobic* exercise (activity that involves abundant motion of the extremities) is beneficial. Many people whose work demands consistent physical activity are fit from doing their work. They are less subject to heart attacks than the remaining 80 percent sedentary segment of our populace.

For those of you who are already at your target weight, it is important that you exercise for heart, lung, and blood vessel benefits. It is unhealthy simply to maintain your weight by consuming the right number of calories to keep you there without also including a sufficient amount of physical activity for your overall well-being. Find an exercise that you like, and incorporate it into your lifestyle. If you are at your desired weight, have not been exercising, and add an activity that is particularly rigorous—say, playing singles tennis every day for an hour (which can burn more than 400 calories)—you will have to add calories to your maintenance level so that you will not lose weight.

Feeling good, being able to enjoy life, and working well are important goals. It is common to have a patient report, after incorporating better living habits, "Doctor, I have never felt this good!" If you are overweight and not sufficiently active—or at your target weight and not sufficiently active—why not incorporate exercise and weight control into your life now and start feeling good *before* having a heart attack, stroke, or other atherosclerotic disease, and reduce your chances of having one? If you are overweight and active, clearly you are not active enough to offset the calories you are consuming, so why not combine your current activity level with cutting calories and reduce your risks, too?

CHAPTER 34

Children, Weight Loss, and Physical Activity

What You Can Do

As you look after your blood vessel and heart health, also think about your children. I urge you to get an early start in helping your children to avoid the problems caused by being overweight and reduce the risk of their getting atherosclerotic diseases later in life. For the same reasons, I also urge you to support your children in being physically active.

Healthy eating habits start in infancy. There is a saying that is worth keeping in mind: "Fat babies become fat children who become fat adults who have heart attacks." It is worth noting, too, that although overweight children continue their tendency to be overweight into adulthood, lean children usually become lean adults. Therefore, babies should not be allowed to become plump.

I disagree with those who oppose reducing calories until a child reaches the age of two years, for fear of interfering with proper development. As long as your child's diet is carefully planned for a healthy balance, eliminating excess calories that produce fat will not reduce the intake of needed nutrients. If your young children are overweight—a problem that occurs with increasing frequency in U.S. society—discuss it with your pediatrician and see what you can do regarding your child's daily diet.

As adults we have the responsibility for our children's well-being until they are adults themselves. Especially if you are the parent of an infant or school-age child, I urge you to act on the following suggestions.

First, feed infants nutritionally. Be sure to consult with your pediatrician about the proper diet and weight for your baby at each stage of his or her growth.

During children's preschool and school years, parents must set a proper example for their children by having healthy eating practices themselves. What hope do children have of not being overweight (and, if already overweight, of losing weight) if they have overweight parents who are unwilling to reform their own unhealthy eating habits?

Parents and concerned community members should utilize the Parent-Teacher Association (PTA) to advocate teaching nutrition in the classroom, starting in kindergarten and continuing through high school. Children of all ages are receptive to this information when it is presented in the context of heart disease. Once, when I was addressing a large school assembly of kindergartners through twelfth graders, I asked all those who had a parent, grandparent, aunt, or uncle who had had a heart attack to raise their hand. More than half of the students raised their hands. When they understood that the topic was real and important, and that it affected their own families, they were extremely interested in learning about nutrition.

Advocate healthy school lunches. Regardless of the size or location of the school, the content of school lunches should be established by professional nutritionists, and parents should be given assurance that this is indeed being carried out. Too frequently, the school lunches served to our children are far too high in carbohydrates. The guidelines I will present in the following chapters for preventing and correcting adult weight excess can also be used as guidelines for school lunches. Again, the PTA is a good forum for discussing this significant topic.

Make sure all soft drink and snack food machines are *absolutely* prohibited in all schools. One twelve-ounce can of cola soda contains 150 calories of sugar, about ten teaspoonfuls. Consuming one such can of soda daily for five days each week will put nearly a pound of fat on your child every four weeks. It is regrettable that some schools permit suppliers to install these machines in exchange for incentives provided by the suppliers. Former president Bill Clinton has started a national movement to accomplish this ban. You can help to initiate local and state legislation to prohibit such machines from public schools. Parents whose children go to private schools have to establish the policy within the schools. The PTA is a good forum for raising this issue, too.

Because physical activity is vital to maintaining a healthy heart and to controlling weight, make sure that physical activity programs in your children's schools involve *all* students, not just children whose athletic skills make them capable of engaging well in competitive sports. School programs should be for physical *conditioning,* not physical competition.

Finally, controlling the weight-generating, excessive caloric consumption of children outside of school is an even greater problem and requires far stronger parental discipline than prevails today. Many chubby children and those on their way to becoming chubby are allowed to consume oversized hamburgers, large servings of french fries, and giant soft drinks. We must not place the entire blame on those who sell these products; they are sold because we buy them. The answer is to stop buying them.

There was a time when a plump baby, and even a plump child, was considered cute. And in fact, despite all that we know about the risks of being overweight, plump babies are still favored and a source of great pride to many mothers and fathers. As a parent, aunt, uncle, or grandparent, you cannot afford to overlook what science tells us about the problems caused by excess weight in babies and young children as well as ourselves. Plumpness is not cute—it is dangerous.

CHAPTER 35

Should You Take Weight-Loss Medications?

Now that I have reminded you about the vital issue of preventing atherosclerosis in your children through diet and exercise, I will return to the subject of your own weight control. I have provided you with an overview of how to create a weight-loss and weight-maintenance system for yourself for heart and blood vessel health. I have explained why I do not recommend low-carb diets and why I advise regular exercise. But it is only human to wonder if there is a shortcut to weight loss. Can I achieve my desired results more quickly? More easily? How about weight-loss medications? The answer to these questions is complicated. The short answer is, *I do not recommend any over-the-counter "food supplement" weight-loss drugs.* Also, you must consult with your doctor about whether prescription medications would actually be helpful to you. The history of weight-loss drugs, both prescribed and over the counter, is fraught with serious problems and even tragedy.

The loudest medical wake-up call in the public news media and in the medical press in recent history was the 1997 explosion of revelations casting doubt on the safety of the highly touted "magic-bullet" weight-loss medications fen-phen and Redux, which had been welcomed by millions of people. These safety concerns led to the U.S. Food and Drug Administration banning the sale of these drugs, which had been the leaders in the multibillion-dollar weight-loss-drug industry.

In 2004, all products containing "herbal" ephedra, a key ingredient in a number of weight-loss products and decongestants, were banned. Ephedra was prominent in the expanding "natural" or "alternative" drug market. It was found to increase heart rates and blood pressure and to cause heart attacks and strokes.

Because some of you may have used one or more of these hazardous drugs and may have sustained ill effects, I want to explain how this alarming sequence of events came about. First, you should know that the above-mentioned weight-loss agents act by altering the amount of chemicals in your brain that influence your appetite. This is a very serious undertaking.

The events leading to the fen-phen epidemic of the 1990s began more than fifty years ago, in the very early years of my practice when the much acclaimed first prescription drugs for weight control, the amphetamines Benzedrine and Dexedrine, were introduced. Though initially quite effective in reducing patients' appetites, it soon became apparent that appetite reduction ceased after a few weeks and blood pressures and heart rates increased. I noticed that some patients began to want their prescriptions refilled early, a sign of overuse and habituation.

Shortly after I stopped prescribing them, the FDA prohibited prescribing these drugs except for a very limited number of conditions. These drugs, originally introduced for weight loss, were the beginning of the street drugs known as "uppers" or "meth."

Seeking safe weight-reduction medications to meet the heavy demand, the pharmaceutical industry set about producing variants of these amphetamines with lesser side effects. One company produced fenfluramine and another phentermine. The FDA approved these for use for periods of a few weeks and with the notation to expect only very limited weight loss. At that time, the FDA had no reason to expect that these two separate drugs, from separate companies, would be used together. However, one doctor who prescribed these medications concluded that if combined, the different brain side effects of the two agents would offset or neutralize each other, and, therefore, they could be combined and used for long periods. At about this time, the FDA approved Redux, a related drug that produced similar actions on the brain. Thus began the famous fen-phen and Redux epidemic. Hundreds of weight-loss clinics were established in the United States, attracting hundreds of thousands of customers. Millions of prescriptions were written.

In 1997 the alarm was sounded with the report that users of these drugs were experiencing an increased frequency of a previously rare disease, primary pulmonary hypertension (PPH), an elevation of the blood pressure in the arteries to the lungs. Some of those affected required surgical lung transplantation. Others died. Soon after, it was learned that numerous users were developing heart valve damage and some required heart valve surgery.

Soon after the fen-phen and Redux problems surfaced, the FDA approved sibutramine, marketed as Meridia. It has actions on brain chemicals similar to those produced by amphetamines. Some advisers opposed approval of this drug because they considered it too risky. Today, use is approved only for patients with severe obesity, and prescribing guidelines exclude use in several conditions, particularly heart and circulatory diseases. An informal survey of pharmacists in my region leads me to believe that it is being prescribed infrequently in this area.

The fen-phen and Redux prohibition left a huge market void for weight-loss medications. This helped herbal "food-supplement" drug sales to flourish, exempt from FDA drug control or approval. Ephedra, of the amphetamine family, is of plant origin and bears the herbal name ma huang. It became the leader in the over-the-counter unlicensed weight-loss-drug preparations until all sales were banned in 2004. Another plant product, Saint-John's-wort, regarded as an antidepressant, affects brain chemicals in a manner similar to the effects of the banned amphetamine fenfluramine. I should note that ephedrine and pseudoephedrine, though chemically related to ephedra and other amphetamine-family drugs I have described, are very respectable medicinal agents and are not implicated in any of the foregoing misadventures. Pseudoephedrine is sold over the counter in the decongestant Sudafed. The sale of this is closely controlled by pharmacies because it can be converted to "meth" drugs, but it has not been found to be involved in producing weight-loss medications.

I will conclude these remarks about "food-supplement" over-the-counter weight-loss products by noting a very disturbing 2004 report by Dr. E. M. Guarneri, a highly respected authority who began her comments with the statement that this topic is one of the most important in cardiology today.[1] This means that it is very important to you! She reported that in 1997, ninety-one million people were using these products. This amounted to 45 percent of the adult population in the United States. Of every five patients taking prescription medications, one was also taking an herbal product, with the risk of potentially dangerous interaction with the prescribed agents. That same year, the year fen-phen and Redux were banned, sales of herbal agents were estimated at $5.1 billion. By 2000, Dr. Guarneri reported that such sales exceeded $8 billion.

My belief is that the 2004 ban of ephedra will attract other products of unknown safety and effectiveness. I urge those of you who are using herbal products to report them to your doctor for advice about their value and safety. I also urge that you report any ill effects you may have experienced from these agents so that your doctor can report this information to the FDA. It was 140 such reports of adverse effects over a period of two years that led to the ban of ephedra. Some of these reports were of heart attacks, strokes, and cardiac arrest, even in young people—a "very scary" situation, according to Dr. Guarneri.

Meanwhile, the pharmaceutical industry has been working to develop safe agents and has produced two that promise to be of value in weight reduction. These products, acarbose and orlistat, have been approved by the FDA as prescription drugs and thus far appear to have merit. They are different from the previously described products that act by influencing the brain chemicals that have to do with appetite control. Instead, acarbose and orlistat interfere with the absorption of starch and fat, respectively. Numerous other weight-loss products are undoubtedly under investigation to meet the huge demand.

CHAPTER 36

Lifesaving Breakthroughs in Drug Treatment for Cholesterol and Triglycerides

In the past two decades, great advances in medications for controlling cholesterols and triglycerides have ushered in an exciting new era in arresting, reversing, and preventing atherosclerosis effectively. These drugs, which include nicotinic acid, the fibrates, the resins, the blockbuster statins, and ezetimibe, drastically reduce heart attacks, strokes, and other blood vessel diseases.

Despite the vital importance of maintaining a proper diet long-term for lipid control, many people rely too heavily on diet alone and delay starting these drugs far too long when they are needed. Do not let this happen to you. If you have heart disease, you must know your cholesterol level. Most of you with an elevation will require a drug to lower it.

We are indebted to the research done over the past fifty years by the AHA, the U.S. government, and pharmaceutical companies to develop lifesaving cholesterol-cutting drugs. The following are the types of medications currently available (more will doubtless be introduced in the future):

1. Nicotinic acid (niacin). This is a natural B-complex vitamin, known for years to reduce cholesterol when taken in very large doses, 1,500 mg to 6,000 mg per day. It reduces cholesterol production in the liver, reducing low-density lipoprotein, increasing high-density lipoprotein, and reducing triglycerides. But there are

certain hazards associated with it that make it infrequently prescribed. I want you to know about it at the beginning of this discussion so that you can be fully informed. One of nicotinic acid's side effects is that it can produce a troublesome, prickly burning-skin sensation. This can usually be prevented by slowly increasing the dose from 100 mg per day to the desired 1,500–6,000 mg and taking an aspirin tablet an hour before the day's first dose. The most serious side effect is liver inflammation, which can be fatal. It is detectable by blood tests at regular intervals that are mandatory for all those taking nicotinic acid. This liver inflammation disappears when the medication is stopped. Slow-release forms of niacin are easier to take, but liver problems are more common, and some doctors refuse to prescribe them. The large doses of nicotinic acid and the liver risks dictate usage only with a doctor's prescription, with regular doctor follow-ups. Although nicotinic acid is inexpensive, its side effects, as mentioned, limit its usage. The volume of over-the-counter sales is a concern. Because of its effect on the liver, this treatment is unsuitable for children.

2. The resins cholestyramine and cholestipol. These powders are taken with food or beverage and, like a magnet, attract cholesterol from the bile in the intestines, carrying it on through the bowels and removing it from the body. They are not absorbed into the circulation and have no side effects except possible constipation and gas. They are excellent agents, reducing LDL by about 20 percent, and are useful in combination with one or more other drugs. Very safe for long-term treatment, they are useful for children and young adults, but statins, described below, may be preferable because they are much more effective in reducing cholesterol.
3. The fibric-acid derivatives gemfibrozil and fenofibrate. These drugs are used chiefly in treating elevated triglycerides. They are sometimes used in conjunction with statins, particularly when there is a combination of high LDL, low HDL, and elevated triglycerides.
4. The statins, the "blockbuster" drugs. Currently there are six on the market—lovastatin, pravastatin, simvastatin, fluvastatin, atorvastatin, and rosuvastatin—with more to come. These are easy to take, with rare side effects (muscle inflammation and liver inflammation, both of which respond to reducing the dose, switching agents, or discontinuing). Statins have reduced heart attacks,

heart attack deaths, strokes, and other atherosclerotic blood vessel diseases. These medications have been tested in more than seventy thousand patients in trials of up to and more than twenty thousand patients each, lasting up to and longer than five years, showing astounding beneficial results in lowering LDL cholesterol levels. They do not, however, correct HDL deficiency. Because so many of you may be taking statins now or may take them in the future, I will briefly discuss details of these trials, which included the following classes of patients:

- those who had had heart attacks and had high cholesterol levels
- those who had had heart attacks and had normal cholesterol levels
- those with high cholesterol who had not had heart attacks or strokes
- people of various ages, extending to as high as eighty
- those with heart disease with a wide range of cholesterol levels from very low to very high

Statins were beneficial in all these groups. Two of these trials have especially exciting results that you should know about.

Discovering What Happens When Statin Dosage Is Increased

As background to understanding these studies, you need to know that for years the federally funded National Cholesterol Education Program has been performing the vital function of establishing normal and abnormal levels, guidelines, and goals in the treatment of cholesterol and other lipid abnormalities. Recommended treatment choices were based on the level of LDL, the presence or absence of other risk factors, and whether the patient had developed coronary heart disease.

The NCEP's 2001 guidelines recommended that patients with known CHD have their LDL reduced by diet or drugs or both to 100 or below. The manufacturer of each of the statins specified the desirable or "standard" dose of each that was needed to reach the goal of reducing LDL by 30 percent to 40 percent and to do this safely. For most but not all of the CHD patients, the standard statin dose brought the LDL down to 100.

Meanwhile, a number of investigators were conducting large studies to determine whether statin doses larger than standard could reduce LDL levels to below 100. They were also conducting studies to see whether these reductions below NCEP guidelines would be of benefit and whether such "high-intensity" dosages would be safe. The results of the treatment trials reported at the time of this writing are startling, and are extremely important to you.

The "Prove It" Trial

In the Prove It study, half of 4,162 patients were treated for twenty-four months with the standard "moderate" 40 mg daily dose of pravastatin.[1] The other half were treated with the "high-intensity" daily dose of 80 mg of atorvastatin. All patients had had a heart attack or "acute coronary syndrome" (severe narrowing that threatens a heart attack), balloon coronary angioplasty, or coronary artery bypass surgery. Treatment was started before hospital discharge, a new feature of this trial since most other such patients had customarily been started on statins only after a trial of diet for months or up to a year, usually showing failure to achieve a desired LDL reduction.

Increased benefits from high-intensity atorvastatin became clear by the end of thirty days. By twenty-four months, the end of the trial, the occurrence of major cardiac events or deaths in the atorvastatin group was 16 percent less than in the pravastatin group. The LDL levels in the former group at the end of twenty-four months averaged 62 versus 95 in the latter. The total cholesterol levels in the atorvastatin group dropped to an average of 130. Tests showed liver inflammation in 3 percent of the high-intensity group as compared with 1 percent in the moderate-dosage group, a small price to pay for the benefits achieved. This trial proved that reducing LDL to below the previously accepted goal of 100 is feasible and beneficial, with acceptable risk. The beneficial results after just thirty days of treatment after acute cardiac emergencies are a strong reason to start statins immediately after such events without the delay of trying diet alone. Although lifelong proper diet is essential in all coronary heart disease patients, those of you with established disease will almost surely require drugs as well. The findings in the following program strengthen this view.

The Reversal Trial

The treatment dosage used in the eighteen-month Reversal study of 502 patients provided the long-sought ability to arrest the progression of coronary atherosclerosis in those with established disease.[2] It also provided the ability to reduce the quantity of cholesterol deposits in the artery walls of such patients. The study findings are among the most significant in the past decade's coronary heart disease research, and they have direct bearing for many of you being treated with statins.

The study was made possible by the remarkable miniaturized ultrasound sensor, or "camera," mounted on the tip of a coronary artery catheter. This instrument recorded for measurement the thickness of the cholesterol deposits in the entire circumference of the artery wall. This permitted calculation of the actual volume or quantity of the deposits.

Measurements of these deposits were made in the 502 patients at the beginning of the study and were repeated during the study and at its termination. Half of the patients were given the standard, moderate daily dose of 40 mg of pravastatin. The other half were given the 80 mg high-intensity daily dose of atorvastatin. Before treatment, both groups had identical levels of LDL, 150 mg. At the end of the study, the pravastatin group had reduced to 110, whereas the atorvastatin patients had reduced to 79, a drop 31 mg greater. More important, whereas the pravastatin patients showed an average increase in cholesterol deposition of 2.7 percent, the atorvastatin patients showed an average reduction of 0.4 percent.

Levels of C reactive protein (an indicator of inflammation anywhere in the body) decreased by 5.2 percent in the pravastatin group compared with 36.4 percent in the atorvastatin patients. This reduction suggests that high-intensity statin treatment reduces inflammation as well as LDL.

The conclusions from the Reversal study are that high-intensity statin therapy can arrest the progression of atherosclerosis and gives promise that regression of existing disease can also be accomplished. If you have experienced a heart attack or have elevated levels of LDL, you can readily see what the long-term benefits of this treatment might be for you.

The NCEP's New Guidelines

The NCEP's guidelines published in 2004 reflect the recent trials that I have just summarized.[3] The following is a summary of some of the guidelines' key features. It will help you to work with your physician in making vital choices that affect your heart and blood vessel health.

Although diet continues to be important in all cases, at certain cholesterol levels, statins should be started at the time of the diet prescription without an initial trial of diet alone. Many such diet trials are now delaying statin therapy by months or up to a year.

Full attention should be given to healthy lifestyle changes, particularly weight control and maintenance of a proper exercise program since they are important approaches to metabolic syndrome. Smoking cessation is crucial.

Attention should be given to "coronary heart disease equivalents" that are now recognized to pose heart attack risks equal to the risks posed by existing coronary artery diseases. These CHD equivalents include atherosclerosis of the leg, abdominal, or carotid arteries and diabetes.

Discovery of CHD of any degree of severity or of any of the CHD equivalents should lead to a decision to start statins. This greatly increases the number of people who are in need of statins.

Although the NCEP guidelines retain the recommendation that all patients with CHD, and now also those with CHD equivalents, should have their LDL reduced to 100 or below, on the basis of recent trials they fully endorse physicians exercising the option of reducing the LDL in such cases to 70.

The NCEP points out that the predictable 30 to 40 percent reduction of LDL cholesterol that the standard statin doses provide may not be sufficient to take the LDL down to the desired level. In such cases, the physician has the option of increasing the statin dose or adding another drug.

The NCEP recommends expanding the use of stains in those who have abnormal cholesterol values but have not developed CHD. Their specific recommendations are based on the level of LDL and the presence or absence of other risk factors. These guidelines will assist your physician in making a treatment decision.

The limitations of statins in treating HDL cholesterol deficiency and triglyceride excess are pointed out. Recommended treatment choices include nicotinic acid and a fibrate used singly or in combination with a statin. Occasional side effects from combining gemfibrozil with a statin have been reduced or eliminated by the recent introduction of fenofibrate.

The 2004 NCEP report's lead author, Dr. Scott Grundy, stated that in 2001 there were estimated to be thirty-six million people in need of drug treatment to lower cholesterol and that the new guidelines would "add a few million."

Concurrent with these advances in statin research and treatment was the companion breakthrough introduction of the "cholesterol absorption inhibitor" ezetimibe.[4] Cholesterol is manufactured in the liver. As a component of bile, it is then discharged into the upper small intestine for absorption into the bloodstream. I mentioned earlier the action of resins in attracting cholesterol like a magnet, then passing it on through the intestines and eliminating it from the body without its entering the bloodstream. This could reduce LDL levels by as much as 20 percent. The absorption inhibitor ezetimibe acts by reducing the passage of cholesterol through the lining of the small intestine into the bloodstream. This results in a substantial reduction in LDL levels, although not to the desired target levels. However, numerous trials have shown that this agent, when given in combination with moderate doses of statins, produces LDL lowering comparable to that produced by the 80 mg high-intensity statin dose. Also, this combined use sometimes reduces LDL to lower levels than were achieved by a single statin regime.

In addition, ezetimibe increases HDL and reduces triglycerides, making it useful in the frequent situation when a person has multiple lipid disorders. Ezetimibe is marketed as a single agent under the name Zetia, which can be used in conjunction with any statin. It is also sold in the highly advertised, very popular Vitorin. This incorporates simvastatin in amounts ranging from 10 mg to 80 mg.

A large two-year study in the Netherlands was completed in 2006 to determine whether combined ezetimibe and simvastatin treatment would slow the progression of atherosclerosis, arrest it, or reduce the volume of cholesterol deposits in carotid arteries.[5] Results of the study have not been reported at the time of this writing, but they are eagerly awaited.

Remember, the medications discussed here reduce heart attacks and strokes, hospitalizations, deaths, and disability. This strongly reinforces my recommendation that each of you establish early in life (or, whatever age you may be, with no delay) an ongoing relationship with a personal physician. Get the necessary tests (see Chapter 37), find out if you need treatment to lower cholesterol and triglycerides, and work out a treatment program with your doctor. The truly lifesaving and disability-reducing advances presented in this chapter are far too important to do otherwise.

Cholesterol Drug Treatment of Children

I have explained that proper diet, with regular exercise, is the foundation of prevention and control of atherosclerosis in children. But because there is such a great risk of this disease in children, the issue of drug treatment of cholesterol and other lipid abnormalities in children and young people is receiving increased attention. (How to identify those children in need of attention is set forth in the next chapter.)

The justifiable concern about possible side effects from long-term use of nicotinic acid has eliminated that drug from consideration for children. Lesser concerns about the side effects of statins and gemfibrozil led to hesitance in using them in children, leaving resins as a safe choice.

The resins pass through the body without absorption and, hence, without risk of systemic effects. However, as a result of the demonstration of the statins' effectiveness and safety in large trials, an increased willingness is emerging to start children on taking the appropriate statins at earlier ages when needed.

My primary purpose here is not to recommend a treatment but to make sure you focus your attention on your children's cholesterol levels and to have them tested. If their levels are abnormal, talk to their doctor about whether he or she thinks they should be treated through diet and exercise alone or with medication, too. The next chapter will teach you the specifics of how to learn whether you and your other family members need to be treated.

CHAPTER 37

Cholesterol and Other Blood Testing

What Tests Should You Have, Where Should You Get Them, and Who Should Administer Them?

By now I am sure you know that everyone should have cholesterol and other blood lipid screenings. The information these tests provide you with is essential for you to make dietary and drug-treatment choices for atherosclerosis and the prevention of atherosclerosis.

What tests are needed? The NCEP guidelines call for performing the basic lipid profiles for everyone at age twenty, with repeat examinations every five years. The basic lipid profiles consist of measuring total cholesterol, LDL, HDL, and triglycerides. If there is a family history of atherosclerotic disease or of blood-lipid abnormality, testing at age two is advised.

Based on my experience with coronary heart disease in very young adults, the high incidence of coronary heart disease observed in young Korean War servicemen,[1] and the frequency of atherosclerosis observed in children in the Bogalusa Heart Study,[2] I strongly disagree with both of these advisories. In the young people whose coronary disease was the subject of the above reports, cholesterol deposits had to begin long before the age of twenty. Testing at age two only those children with a positive family history will leave out many children who need to be tested. As mentioned, although grandparents of children aged two will likely have been diagnosed if they have coronary disease, coronary heart disease may not yet have been diagnosed in parents, aunts, and uncles, even if it is present.

Following current guidelines prevents some children from being identified as possibly having inherited risk. It is also important to realize that some children may develop cholesterol abnormalities at an early age even if they do not have a family history of it. I strongly advocate that carrying out the basic lipid profile be a mandatory preschool requirement for all children. I also believe that all children with normal values at age two be retested at puberty.

In reviewing the basic lipid profile for children, bear in mind the lower levels of normal in youngsters. *Total cholesterol should be no higher than 140 to 160.* Any level 170 or above before the age of seventeen is considered abnormal.

As mentioned, in view of the exciting new information about arresting and, I hope, regressing coronary atherosclerosis, adults need to be regularly tested. Each of you needs to know exactly where you stand in respect to all your risks. Cholesterol and triglyceride measurements should be a part of your first checkup with your doctor. If they are not, request the tests. Ask your doctor for a report of the level of each lipid component and maintain your own written record of the exact numbers your test showed; it is not enough to be told, "Your tests are okay."

What tests do you need? As mentioned, you need the basic lipid profile (total cholesterol, LDL and HDL cholesterol, and triglyceride levels). This requires a twelve-hour fast prior to testing.

Adding a fasting blood-sugar level to the tests is increasingly regarded as important to detect diabetes. In addition to the fasting sugar level, a two-hour level after consuming a sugar-containing beverage is considered even more accurate. Even better as an indicator of diabetes is a "glucose-tolerance test," with hourly blood-sugar measurements for three to five hours after a sweetened beverage.

I have mentioned a harmful component of LDL known as subclass B (also known as "small dense LDL particles"). This is high on the growing list of factors that are being identified with the inception and progression of atherosclerosis and also can be tested for. Correction of subclass B LDL may require a different treatment from that usually employed to reduce LDL as a whole. Another lipoprotein, "LP(a)", which I have also mentioned, and which can be tested for too, is inherited and has adverse effects that are currently being studied.

In addition to these lipoproteins, authorities are drawing attention to two other substances they have identified as emerging risk factors. They are fibrinogen and C reactive protein. Homocysteine excess (see Chapter 14), though at present not considered a risk factor, is associated with heart disease.

For easy reference, here are the Mayo Clinic Laboratories' recommendations for testing:

- Lipid panel (total, HDL, and LDL cholesterols and triglycerides)
- Lipoprotein (a)
- LDL subclass fractionation
- Fibrinogen
- C reactive protein
- Homocysteine

Your doctor can have blood drawn for these tests, but some of the tests may not be available at your local hospital. If this is the case, blood samples may be taken, and your local hospital (known as the referring hospital) may then ship the samples to another hospital (the reference lab) for analysis. When the Mayo Clinic performs the analysis, as it does for hospitals in Springfield, its report to the referring hospital includes an informative risk summary of the substances tested for and treatment comments. All of this would be of value to you and your doctor.

Which of these tests besides the basic lipid panel should you have? Opinions vary. It is generally agreed that everyone with a family history of heart attack, stroke, leg artery disease, or thrombophlebitis at an early age (especially under age forty) has the possibility of elevated LDL subclass B or lipoprotein (a) levels. These are not disclosed by the basic lipid panel. Everyone who is taking cholesterol- or triglyceride-lowering medication and who is not responding promptly and decisively should also have more extensive tests. So should everyone who has atherosclerotic disease if conventional testing has revealed only minimal risk from the substances reported on in the basic lipid panel.

The possible importance of testing for emerging risk factors was driven home to me personally when the Mayo Extended Risk Panel showed that a member of my family has a very high level of C reactive protein, previously undetected. Testing for the identified and emerging risk factors will tell you what treatment and lifestyle changes you need to make to improve your heart and blood vessel health.

What about testing for homocysteine? Although future research will tell us homocysteine's role, if any, in heart disease, at present we know that excess homocysteine is associated with heart and other atherosclerotic diseases. When it appeared that homocysteine was a risk factor, testing for it was advisable because an excess could be corrected with B vitamins and folic acid. Currently, homocysteine excess can be considered only an indication that risk of heart and other atherosclerotic diseases is present. At this time, my opinion is that testing for homocysteine excess is optional, and you should discuss it with your doctor.

Two barriers may stand in the way of getting the more extensive testing. The first is the high cost of these tests, which may or may not be covered by insurance carriers. Some regard certain of these tests as valuable only for research, an opinion with which I disagree. Since the tests are being increasingly discussed in medical circles, insurance carriers will probably approve more of them. Your doctor's protests to insurance carriers will also help. The second obstacle to getting these special blood tests is simply not knowing about them. I have described them in this chapter so that this will not be a problem for you. As I have said before, physicians appreciate and respect the wishes of highly informed patients, so you must not hesitate to speak out with your questions and requests.

For easy reference, here is a summary of my recommendations for blood screening:

- Essential: total, LDL, and HDL cholesterols and triglycerides—minimum twelve-hour fast required (total cholesterol and total LDL and HDL cholesterol are not adequate)
- At your doctor's discretion, requiring special order, testing for:
  1. LDL subclass
  2. Lipoprotein (a)
  3. C reactive protein
  4. Fibrinogen level
  5. Blood-sugar levels
  6. Homocysteine level

I have also prepared Appendix A, "Laboratory Tests for Cardiovascular Risk," to enhance your knowledge of the tests, their availability, and their costs. I mentioned that Springfield hospitals use reference labs such as the Mayo Clinic. Ordering the Mayo Clinic's Extended Risk Panel is convenient for your hospital, requiring a single transmission of blood specimen. As of this writing, the Mayo's charge for the package is less than four hundred dollars, similar to the sum of approximate charges listed in Appendix A. As mentioned, so far insurance coverage for this is uncertain, but if it is disallowed under the category of "research purposes only," you can file a protest, as can your physician.

What about tests outside your doctor's office? Increasing recognition of the need for cholesterol testing has led to a variety of public screening programs by hospitals, civic organizations, and pharmacies. Home-testing kits are also available. The question is if such tests have value.

These testing programs are carried out in one of two ways. Most employ the traditional method of testing a blood specimen obtained from an arm vein. This sample is then taken to a traditional laboratory supervised by a physician. Results are reported by mail or telephone to the person who was tested. The other method is to examine a drop of blood obtained by finger-stick (a quick jab of a needle into the tip of the finger), with an immediate report. A number of devices have been developed to do this type of testing. Some are used at locations such as pharmacies, and some are for home use. The capability of this equipment ranges from producing only a total cholesterol report to producing a full basic lipid profile and blood-sugar level. Some home units provide kits for performing only two tests; others provide for multiple tests. Clearly, home kits and finger-jab tests at the pharmacy do not provide you with the full testing you need and should not be used as a substitute for screenings by a doctor.

Public screenings—blood tests performed at shopping malls and public events—have advantages and disadvantages. On the plus side, these programs attract some people who are not affiliated with a personal physician and who may be prompted by possibly abnormal test results to engage a doctor. But they also present many disadvantages.

The accuracy of some testing is subject to question, particularly tests using finger-stick blood specimens. If this method is chosen (whether in a public screening or at home), check to make sure that the device and service bear the endorsement of a recognized authority because otherwise it will not even have validity, even for the limited tests performed. Additionally, in public screenings the number of tests carried out may be inadequate, ranging from total cholesterol level only to the basic lipid panel consisting of total, LDL, and HDL cholesterols and triglyceride levels, sometimes with blood sugar added.

Such test results should be viewed in the context of your overall condition, including other risk factors. There is no one at a public screening to do this. Another disadvantage is the very real drawback that being given test results that are considered normal by the person giving you the report—who may not be well trained—may falsely reassure you about your total condition. This may cause you to be less inclined to engage a personal physician when, in fact, it may be essential for you to do so. All of this means that there is no substitute for a personal physician.

CHAPTER 38

Should You Take Aspirin Regularly?

As you probably know, ordinary aspirin has the ability to interfere with the clumping of blood platelets, which reduces their ability to form blood clots. *This is why I have advised that if you think you are experiencing an early warning sign of a heart attack, you should immediately chew a full-size uncoated aspirin.* In view of the plethora of aspirin advertisements telling you to take aspirin regularly to prevent a heart attack, you need to know whether this advice is sound.

Recently, noted cardiology researcher Dr. Valentin Fuster addressed the question, "Who should take aspirin and how much?" Fuster described aspirin as "a miracle drug" and said that anyone who has experienced an atherosclerotic disease—a heart attack, stroke, or disease of the carotid or peripheral arteries—should be on it. "In those sustaining a heart attack or an acute coronary syndrome or [who] have had coronary artery bypass surgery," he explained, taking aspirin means "the risk of later events is reduced by 20 to 25 percent."[1] However, Fuster points outs that 10 to 25 percent of people are resistant to these positive effects of aspirin and that it is difficult to identify people with this resistance.

What if you have not had a coronary disease? Should you take aspirin regularly? According to Fuster, if you have not had a coronary disease, you should not take aspirin as a preventive measure unless you have two or more risk factors (see Chapter 11).

For those for whom aspirin is recommended, Fuster says the dosage should be 80 to 160 mg, with a one-time initial dose of 325 mg. So if you have an established atherosclerotic disease or two or more risk factors, consult with your doctor about what your aspirin dosage should be.

CHAPTER 39

Why Smoking Causes Heart Attacks and Strokes—and How I Stopped Smoking

If you smoke, you already know you should stop. Billboards and public service announcements tell you to stop; family and friends tell you to stop. You know that smoking is a cause of lung cancer. However, you may not know what makes smoking one of the "big three" risks for heart attacks and one of the major risks of strokes. The reason for this is that in the act of smoking, the intake of nicotine (which is contained in all tobacco) can cause a spasm, a narrowing or constriction of blood vessels interfering with passage of blood through those vessels. This narrowing can create or contribute to the complete obstruction of an artery and thus cause a heart attack or stroke. (Smoking also increases the risk of hypertension, the subject of the next chapter.)

This is not a scientific treatise on how to stop smoking, but I hope it will help those of you who find yourself still smoking. It is a personal and professional tale of my own nicotine addiction and how sharing the way that I stopped smoking helped many of my patients to stop, too.

Since so many people begin smoking in adolescence, and undoubtedly many of you are in the position to influence the children around you, I will start my story in my own teenage years. I started college at fifteen, and found that I was the youngest freshman in school. My classmates called me "the kid." Always too small to successfully compete in sports and on the playground, I desperately sought to be "one of the guys" in college. I thought that taking up smoking would show that I was a man. Although that did not work to impress people as I had hoped it would, I continued smoking while I concentrated on doing well academically.

At first I rolled my own cigarettes with R. J. Reynolds sack tobacco. Next I used a cigarette-rolling device, then graduated to Wings, the ten-cents-a-pack economy brand of cigarettes, before winding up with a pack a day of Lucky Strikes.

It did not take long after I started my medical practice to realize that smoking was very bad for my heart and lung patients. I realized I had to stop smoking for my own sake and to set an example for them, but I was genuinely addicted, and several attempts showed me that stopping "cold turkey" was impossible. During the attempts, I would often hide out to smoke so those around me would not observe my failure.

My answer came from a magazine article. The method the article suggested was simple. It consisted of making a decision to reduce smoking by one cigarette per day, with the understanding that it was okay to sometimes take two or three days to get down another cigarette. I carried an index card to record the time of each smoke, and my total number of cigarettes for the day. When I was down to my last cigarette, I sat for two hours looking at it before deciding not to smoke it. The entire process of stopping took only a few weeks.

My patients and I maintained a very friendly discourse about smoking. Few patients failed to stop. I never criticized a patient for smoking. We talked about the improvements in breathing and the lessening of coughing that occur when smoking is stopped. We also talked about the financial benefits, money savings that could contribute significantly to household budgets or special presents for yourself or for your family.

At the same time as I was giving up smoking I was also dealing with my weight problem. After removing smoke irritation from my mouth, I was pleased to learn that my sense of taste improved so much that I was satisfied with a smaller amount of food. This taught me that it is incorrect to assume that stopping smoking will automatically cause you to gain weight.

Word of my patients' and my success in stopping smoking brought many invitations for me to speak publicly about this vital topic to heart health. Years later I acquired a valuable punch line about the "eight-minute cigarette." A study came out showing that a smoker's life is shortened by eight minutes for each cigarette smoked. Even more impressive was a forty-year study of thirty-four thousand male British doctors reported in 1994 showing that those who smoked had shorter lives of six and a half years on average. This amounted to an average of eleven minutes for each cigarette smoked.[1]

I continued supporting patients in the practice of cutting down one cigarette per day (or per two or three days) throughout my career. The introduction of nicotine skin patches helped most of my patients who continued to smoke. I prescribed these exclusively rather than less effective measures such as nicotine gum and oral medications.

I agree with those who say that nicotine addition is equivalent to heroin addiction. I cannot conceive of a heroin addict kicking the habit alone. Therefore, I strongly believe that you should involve your doctor in your program to stop smoking. If your doctor is not supportive and interested in helping, I recommend that you seek someone who is.

And again, while you are improving your own health through stopping smoking, make sure your children never start. If your child's school does not teach children the dangers of smoking, advocate creating a program to do so.

CHAPTER 40

Blood Pressure Control

A Neglected Medical Milestone

Of the "big three" risks for heart attack—cholesterol or triglyceride excess or both, smoking, and hypertension (high blood pressure)—the easiest to correct is hypertension. Yet many people in need of the lifesaving treatment available for hypertension do not receive it. What makes this worse is that high blood pressure is not only one of the big three risks for a heart attack but also the number-one risk for a stroke.

Why don't more people get treatment? There are three reasons. First, most people have not yet become sufficiently aware of the problem and the benefits available from treatment. Second, doctors have not yet become sufficiently committed to initiating treatment and assuming a long-term follow-up partnership with patients to guarantee continuity of treatment. And third, "managed-care" health plans, which bear the cost of much of today's ongoing preventive patient care, require limiting physician time per patient. Hypertension management requires generous physician attention. Thus, the crucial time needed for diagnosis, treatment, and continuing follow-up is being shortened by decree of the paying authority. This situation deserves your outcry!

Do not wait to discover whether you have high blood pressure by experiencing a stroke or other negative consequence. Ask your physician if his or her time availability will permit full, continuing attention to blood pressure as well as attention to lipids and other risks on a long-term basis. If not, and if it is your physician's choice rather than the managed-care system's policy that is causing the problem, get a referral to another physician. It is widely known that many patients who start on hypertension medication are not taking it a year later. In my experience, patients' inattention to this serious problem can be corrected only through a strong, lasting patient-physician partnership.

If your managed-care system does not allow ongoing tests and care for hypertension, register a complaint and keep complaining until you get the necessary change. In the meantime, go to a physician outside of your managed-care system to get a blood pressure test, and discuss the results with that physician. This should not be too expensive. If you need treatment, you may be able to find a way to work with your managed-care primary physician, and, if necessary, a physician consultant outside of the managed-care network.

For easy reference, see the table of blood pressure levels (remember that systolic refers to the peak pressure reached following a heartbeat and diastolic refers to the lowest pressure between heartbeats):

Causes and Treatments

Except in a very small percentage of cases where high blood pressure is brought about by kidney disease or adrenal gland tumors, to this day nobody knows exactly what causes hypertension. But here is what you should know about treatment: it may save your life!

Effective treatment of hypertension began in the early 1950s. It has been a delight and a privilege to see this formerly deadly disease become controllable and thereby abruptly decrease the number of patients dying from heart attacks, strokes, and congestive heart failure.

The first drug of value for treating the predominant form of high blood pressure, essential hypertension—the cause of which is still unknown—was reserpine. Reserpine is an extract from the snakeroot (rauwolfia) plant of India and has tranquilizing power. It is said that Mahatma Ghandi maintained emotional composure by constantly chewing snakeroot.

Table 40.1.
Normal and abnormal blood pressures

Normal

Systolic: 100 to 140 MM (130-39 is borderline high)

Diastolic: 60 to 90 MM (80-89 is borderline)

Examples
Normal: 120/80
Borderline: 135/85

Elevated

Systolic: Above 140 MM

Diastolic: Above 90 MM

Examples
150/95, 170/110, 180/130

Elevation of systolic pressure alone

150 MM or above

Examples
160/80, 180/85, 190/82

Note: MM = millimeters of mercury.

Hexamethonium came next. This was an agent that chemically paralyzed or blocked the sympathetic (autonomic) nerves, which regulate our blood pressure, reducing blood pressure to the desired level. Hexamethonium could bring malignant hypertension to a halt—a near miracle—and could provide maintenance control of the more common essential hypertension.

Next were the highly effective thiazide diuretics. Diuretics function by eliminating sodium from the body through the urine. Thiazide diuretics include chlorthiazide (Diuril), hydrochlorothizide (Hydrodiuril), and chlorthalidone, which many of you are probably taking because currently it has proven to be the best. These medications revolutionized the treatment of hypertension. They were also indispensable in the lifesaving elimination of excess body fluids in congestive heart failure.

Later, the beta-blockers, propanolol and others, were introduced. These block much of the action of norepinephrine in elevating the blood pressure and also help to control rapid heart rates and rhythm irregularities.

Calcium-channel blockers followed and soon became frequent first-choice drugs in hypertension management.

Last introduced were two classes of drugs with similar effects, the ACE inhibitors and the angiotension receptor blocker. These have also proved valuable after a heart attack and in congestive failure.

After previously focusing on reducing the diastolic blood pressure elevation (the minimum reached between heartbeats), research has recently shown great value in reducing the systolic blood pressure. It was found that this, too, could be effectively treated.

Revolutionary news came in a 2002 report of the results in 33,357 patients with hypertension, comparing six years of treatment with three commonly used drugs.[1] The conclusion: "Thiazide-type diuretics are superior in preventing one or more major forms of cardiovascular disease and are less expensive. This should be preferred for first-step antihypertension therapy." The thiazide tested was chlorthalidone, available for decades at a very low cost compared with the expensive, more recently introduced calcium-channel blockers and ACE inhibitors. Diuretic use decreased dramatically with the advent of these latter medications. If people had continued using the earlier diuretics instead of changing to the more costly medications, there would have been a savings of $3.1 billion!

Many patients with hypertension will require more than one drug, even as many as three or four. If a diuretic such as chlorthalidone is not completely effective, the more expensive medications can be added. Doing this is a cost-efficient as well as medically sound approach.

Excessive sodium intake from sodium chloride, either in food processing, in cooking, or as table salt, can cause or worsen hypertension. Excess salt use is almost universal. Total usage per day should not exceed 6 grams (2,400 milligrams of sodium), and in some cases should be far less. Discuss your optimum level of salt intake with your doctor. Learn to read food-content labels and use no salt or less salt in cooking and at the table. The amount of alcohol consumed also contributes to hypertension, and, if excessive, may have to be reduced.

During the decades of drug development for treating hypertension, it was ultimately recognized that weight excess and physical inactivity were contributory causes of hypertension in a significant percentage of patients. It was also discovered that for many, correction of these problems could correct the hypertension. These findings were a crucial factor in generating the concept of changing your lifestyle to improve your health, an approach that, as you know, is important in other aspects of treatment, too, particularly lipid control and diabetes prevention.

Concurrent with these developments were studies showing that other infrequent causes of hypertension were kidney and adrenal gland diseases. It was soon learned that if the causative kidney problem affected only one kidney, surgical removal of that kidney cured the hypertension. Later it was found that narrowing or blockage of the renal artery (the vessel carrying blood to the kidney) was often the cause of the kidney (or renal) hypertension. This led to bypass grafting, surgical removal of the obstructing atheroma, or balloon angioplasty with or without stent placement to correct this condition.

Discovery of the diseases of the adrenal glands, which produce the norepinephrine causing the hypertension, also led to surgical remedies. One was removal of the rare adrenal gland tumor pheochromocytoma to cure the hypertension. The other surgical cure was removal of portions of the overactive adrenal glands.

Although the relationship between stress and hypertension has not yet been precisely defined, research on reducing mild to moderate hypertension through relaxation techniques, meditation, cognitive behavioral techniques (learning new ways to deal with stress), biofeedback, yoga, and tai chi has shown positive results. Some studies report not only that these alternative methods have lowered patients' blood pressure but that using them on a continuing basis can also maintain reduced blood pressure with a lower dose of medication, and, in some cases, no medication at all.[2] Talk to your doctor about combining these approaches with medication and testing to see what effect they have on your blood pressure and your medication dosage.

All of this is good news. It means that today, through medications, diet, and other treatment methods, virtually all cases of hypertension can be controlled, even though only a few are curable. It is a sad fact, however, that many of you reading this book do not even know you have hypertension, since it produces no symptoms until a possibly devastating consequence occurs. Others of you may not have adequate treatment or may have stopped taking your medications because you became complacent after having good blood pressure for a few months.

This one issue is reason enough for you to have an ongoing, year-after-year relationship with your physician. Although public screenings and home blood pressure measuring devices can help determine whether you have hypertension, you need more than that. Even if your pressure is normal, you need to know if you have other risks and if, over time, your pressure gradually rises to a level requiring treatment. This requires regular testing by, and discussion with, your personal physician.

Nevertheless, the excellent, inexpensive, home blood pressure measuring devices have an important function in your relationship with your physician: they can identify a condition known as "white coat hypertension," which makes your blood pressure rise only when you are in the company of your doctor. Home blood pressure measuring devices can also help you identify significant elevations during stressful situations outside the doctor's office. You need to make sure that readings with your machine agree with those in the doctor's office. If they do not, discuss it with your doctor. You owe it to yourself to take this chapter to heart.

CHAPTER 41

What Every Woman Should Know about Coronary Disease in Women

Until recently, heart attacks have been presumed to be a malady of men, but today most people recognize that they equally affect women. In fact, coronary disease is the number-one cause of death in women after menopause, accounting for half the deaths, 230,000 to 250,000 per year. Heart and circulatory diseases, chief among which is the heart attack, cause twice as many deaths as all cancers combined and ten times as many as breast cancer.[1]

Although menopause, natural or surgical, quadruples the heart attack risk, premenopausal women are not exempt. Notwithstanding hormone protection at this age through maintenance of higher levels of high-density lipoprotein (that is, HDL, or "good," cholesterol) than occur in men, and greater control of low-density lipoprotein (LDL, or "bad," cholesterol), women can be at increased risk at any age in the following ways:

- Smoking (24 percent of women smoke, more than ever before, increasing heart attacks two- to sixfold).
- Adding birth-control pills to smoking enormously increases risk.
- Hypertension enhances risk—half of the women who have heart attacks have high blood pressure.
- Lack of exercise enhances risk—and few women get adequate exercise.

* Diabetes quadruples risk.
* Weight excess enhances risk. Weight gain, usually starting early in adulthood, advances insidiously, and its risks have only recently been appreciated, increasing heart deaths as follows:[2]

11–17 lbs. excess	25 percent increase
18–23 lbs. excess	64 percent increase
24–42 lbs. excess	92 percent increase
43 lbs. and above excess	165 percent increase

At menopause, as a result of the hormonal changes, the level of good cholesterol drops and that of bad cholesterol increases. One out of three women then develops cholesterol excess, averaging 240 to 260 by age fifty-five. Triglycerides also increase—indeed, triglycerides increase more in women at this age than in men.

Lowering cholesterol after menopause markedly reduces coronary disease. The question is how you accomplish this effectively. Although diet and exercise are the means of eliminating risk from weight excess, cholesterol control after menopause by diet alone is very disappointing. It is often, if not usually, necessary to add medication; statins reduce coronary risk by a reported 29 percent.

Much discussion is taking place about whether there is merit in reversing the estrogen hormone deprivation of menopause by replacement therapy. The lower incidence of coronary disease in women before menopause than in men of the same age has been attributed to estrogen maintaining HDL at a higher level and LDL at a lower level. Therefore, it seemed logical to restore those protective levels after menopause by administering hormones. There are the additional factors that resumption of hormones is believed to be beneficial to the lining (endothelium) of the coronary arteries, producing a desirable blood vessel–dilating effect and reducing the arteries' ability to form blood clots.

Because of the unproven assumption that these benefits actually occurred, and because of known noncardiac benefits from hormone use (such as simply feeling better, being relieved of hot flashes, and reduced aging of the skin), millions of women were being prescribed hormone replacement therapy on a long-term basis. Spurred by the increasing interest in and concern about coronary disease in women, authorities wisely concluded it was necessary to determine whether long-term hormone administration is appropriate. This led to studies of many thousands of women with and without coronary disease, comparing hormone treatments with placebo (no treatment) over periods of years. It was surprising and very disappointing that these huge trials failed to show coronary disease benefit from hormone treatment after menopause and indicated the occurrence of some adverse cardiovascular and other effects. Discussions and some debate about these startling results continue, so it is not possible to offer here what might amount to recommendations about hormone use. This advice must come from your physician.

Because of hormonal differences between women and men, heart attacks in women most frequently occur ten or more years later than in men, unless there are premenopausal high-risk factors that lead to an early heart attack. Overall, women have as many heart attacks as men; the fact that women live longer is due in part to women's heart attacks occurring at a later age.

Notwithstanding the increasing recognition of the high incidence of coronary heart disease in women, studies show that on average women are slower than men to respond to the heart attack early warning signs, are less frequently diagnosed accurately and promptly, are less intensively tested and treated, and have higher death rates after sustaining heart attacks. This unfortunate sequence is generally attributed to the prevailing opinion that heart attack symptoms in women are different from those in men and thus are not recognized as quickly as are men's symptoms. It is often said that heart attack symptoms in women are "atypical" in contrast with the classic "crushing chest pain" of men. Both assertions are incorrect: women's symptoms are not atypical, and, as you know from earlier chapters, men do not always experience "crushing chest pain" as a symptom of a heart attack.

I do not know of any studies comparing the frequency of specific heart attack symptoms in women with those in men, but, based on my experience with thousands of patients, I have observed that heart attack symptoms in women and men are similar. Part of the reason for the confusion about women having different symptoms is that up to now the full array of early warning signs has been very inadequately taught to both women and men. Correcting this is one of the primary purposes of this book!

Remember that, as noted in Part I, a study of 460,000 men and women who sustained heart attacks showed that 33 percent of them had no chest pain or discomfort. Remember, too, that if chest discomfort appears, at first it is usually mild, possibly intermittent, which is why it is wrong to think that women may experience chest discomfort, whereas for men crushing chest pain is "classic." In fact, as I have explained, crushing chest pain occurs in some people and not in others. The symptoms that have been incorrectly called atypical are actually what I have identified in Chapter 3 as the "little-known signs of a heart attack." These symptoms are typical; the problem is that they are frequently unrecognized and ignored by the people experiencing them. Slow recognition by health professionals in the emergency room is also frequent, delaying and reducing the intensity of treatment.

For both women and men, some of the common descriptions of symptoms that need modification include the following. Arm discomfort is usually described as being in the left arm rather than in either the right or left arm or both, and is sometimes described as numbness rather than pain. Neck and jaw pain is sometimes low down in the list of symptoms—it should be at the top of the list along with chest and arm discomfort. Upper abdominal discomfort is usually inadequately described as "indigestion" or "stomach pain." Sweating, usually low on the list of symptoms, should be moved up on a par with shortness of breath—and it should not be described as a "cold sweat" but rather simply as sweating without apparent cause. "Sudden weakness" is more accurate than "fatigue," the word often used to describe a lack of energy that may precede a heart attack. The key to weakness being a symptom of a heart attack is that it is sudden—it is not a chronic condition, and it often appears all at once and not as a consequence of physical exertion.

Thus, again for both genders, the early warning signs of a heart attack—including the little-known early warning signs—are:

- Discomfort in the center of the chest—
  - pressure
  - fullness
  - squeezing
  - aching
  - burning
- possibly extending into one or both arms, the neck, jaws, upper abdomen, or back. It may occur in any one or all these areas without being in the front of the chest.

- Also possibly present—
  sweating
  shortness of breath
  nausea
  sudden weakness

If you experience any of these warning signs, call your doctor, if possible, or get to your emergency room by the quickest available means.

A great deal of investigation is being conducted to determine why the death rate in women after heart attacks, even if optimally treated, is slightly higher than in men. Part of this study concerns the question of whether the smaller diameter of coronary arteries in women than in men of larger build is somehow responsible.

I am certain that this chapter has made more firm in your mind the importance of knowing the early warning signs and promptly responding if any of them occur, regardless of your gender.

CHAPTER 42

Health, Awareness, and Lifestyle

From the first page of this book you have been learning how to recognize, treat, and prevent heart attacks and strokes, major causes of death and disability in the United States and around the world. In the Introduction I mentioned that some of you may initially find this information scary, because you would prefer not to think about illness at all. But as I have shown you, in this case the information can be lifesaving. With regard to heart attacks and strokes, ignorance is not just dangerous; it can be lethal.

We live in a time in which treatment of heart attacks and strokes is better than ever before. Breakthroughs have made it possible for early recognition and treatment in some cases to prevent damage from occurring, and in other cases to limit it. We also live in a time in which knowledge about and medications to assist in prevention provide unprecedented opportunities for reducing the risk. This is wonderful news for all of us.

I hope you can see from reading this book that if you do not already have a healthy lifestyle, starting today you can take steps to create one for yourself. You can eliminate unhealthy eating practices and, without a lot of complication and stress, learn how to eat more healthily with a practical, doable, enjoyable system of choosing food that you can create yourself. You can increase your level of exercise without having to become an expert on heart rates or do anything more complicated or costly than taking a walk near your home or your office or on a treadmill. You can have regular checkups with a personal physician to assess and monitor conditions that might cause you problems later and that frequently can be corrected through proper treatment or changes in lifestyle. In doing this, you are not only increasing your chances of living longer but also increasing your quality of life—your ability to be fully alive and productive.

Appendix A

Laboratory Tests for Cardiovascular Risk

Test	Availability	Cost
Lipid profile—initial exam Total cholesterol, LDL cholesterol HDL cholesterol, triglycerides	All hospitals, private local labs, public screenings, pharmacy screenings	$ 23
LDL subclass gradient GEL electrophoresis	Reference and research labs	85
HDL subclass gradient GEL electrophoresis	Reference and research labs	120
LP(a)	Reference labs	20-50
APO A	Reference labs	26
APO B	Reference labs	26
APO C-H	Research labs	——
APO E-2, -3, -4 typing	Reference labs	33
Fasting blood glucose	All hospital and local labs	7
Glucose tolerance	All hospital and local labs	22
Insulin level	Reference labs	50
Homocysteine level	Large hospital labs	25-50
Fibrinogen level	Most hospital labs	15
C reactive protein level	Reference labs	124

Sources: Private, hospital, and reference labs; Medicare reimbursement schedules.

Note: The assistance of Dr. Lori Wilson, St. John's Regional Health Center, Springfield, Missouri, is appreciated.

Appendix B

Recommended Dietary Allowances of Vitamins

Vitamin	Males	Females			Proposals
		Adult	Pregnancy	Lactation	
A	5,000 IU[a]	4,000 IU	5,000 IU	6,000 IU	
B_1	1.2-1.5 mg[b]	1.0-1.1 mg	1.5-1.6 mg	1.5-1.6 mg	
B_2	1.7-1.8 mg	1.2-1.3 mg	1.7-1.8 mg	1.7-1.8 mg	
B_3	15-19 mg	13-15 mg	18-20 mg	18-20 mg	
B_5	10 mg	10 mg	10 mg	10 mg	
B_6[c]	2 mg	1.6 mg	2.1 mg	2.1 mg	
B_{12}[c]	6 mcg[d]	6 mcg	6 mcg	6 mcg	
C[e]	60 mg	60 mg	70 mg	90-95 mg	
D	400 IU to age 24 200 IU after 24	400 IU to age 24 200 IU after 24	400 IU	400 IU	
E[e]	30 IU	30 IU	30 IU	30 IU	
Folic acid[c]	200 mcg	180 mcg	400 mcg	280 mcg	400- 2,000 IU

[a]IU = international units

[b]mg = milligram

[c]Reducer of homocysteine (also has other functions)

[d]mcg = microgram

[e]Antioxidant vitamin (also has other functions)

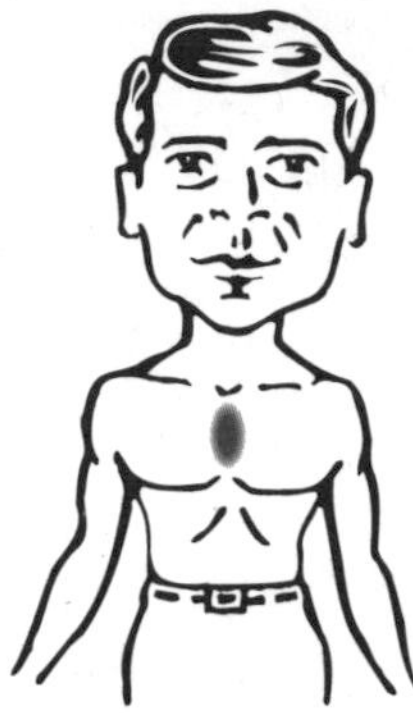

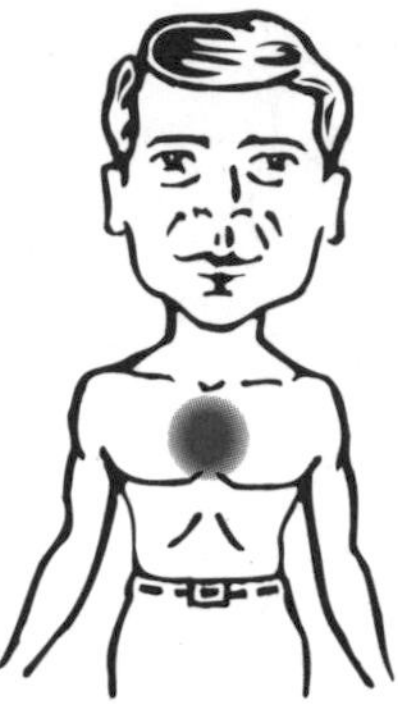

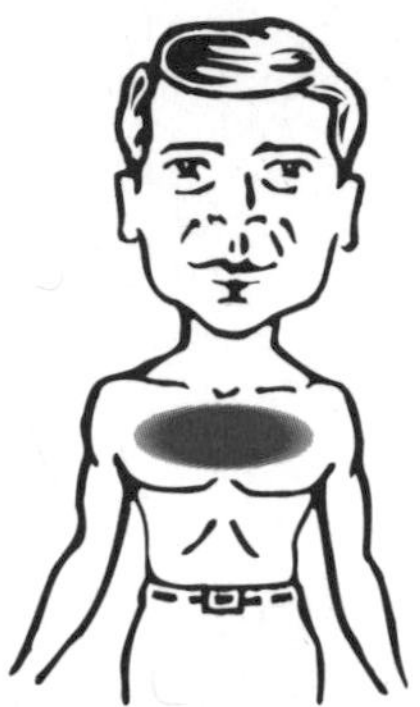

Most heart pain occurs as a sensation of pressure, fullness, squeezing, or aching in the center of the chest, "under the necktie." It may be mild, moderate, or severe, radiating through the whole chest, but it is usually not a sharp, jabbing type of pain.

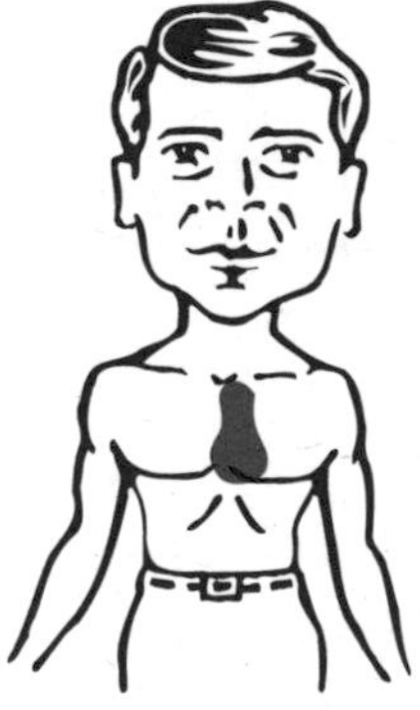

The heart is in the center of the chest, not on the left, as many people believe.

THE EARLY WARNING SIGNS

Discomfort in the center of the chest—

- **Pressure**
- **Fullness**
- **Squeezing**
- **Aching**
- **Burning**

—possibly extending into one or both arms, the neck, jaws, upper abdomen, or back. It may occur in any one or all these areas without being in the front of the chest area.

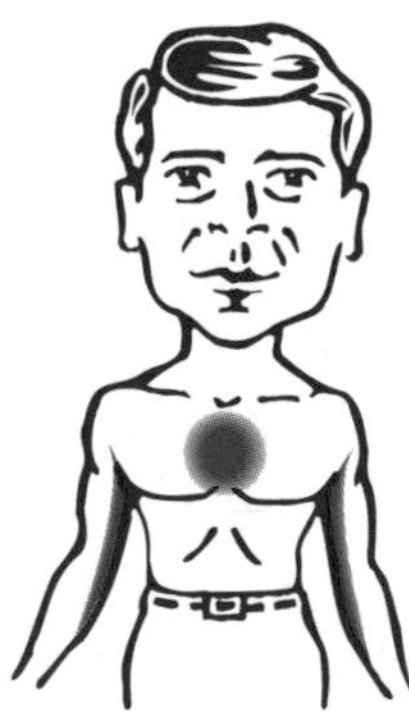

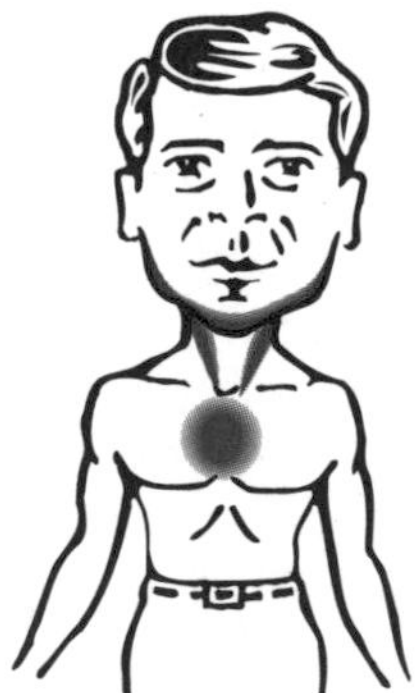

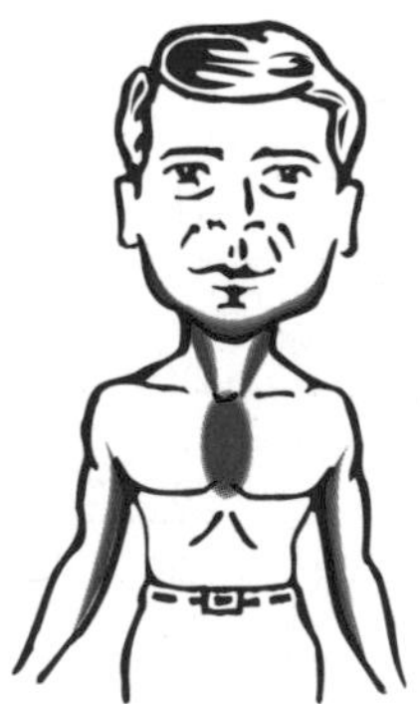

Common combinations of pain are chest and one or both arms; chest and neck or jaws; or all possible areas, including the upper abdomen. Sweating, shortness of breath, nausea, or vomiting may occur. With any of these pains, call a doctor or get to a hospital fast!

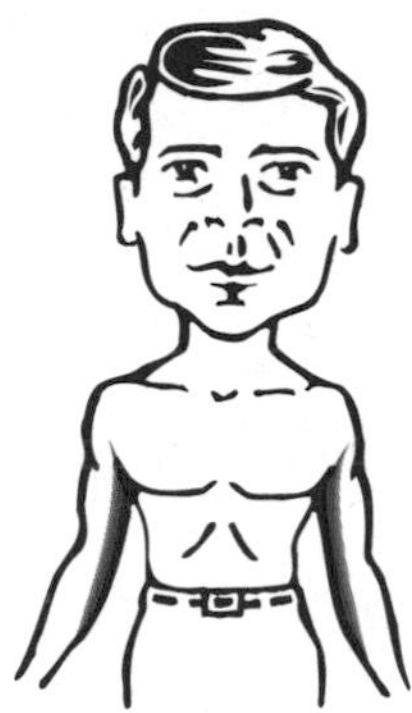
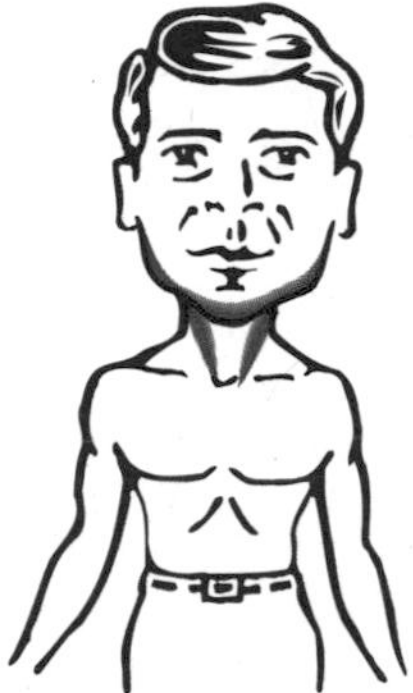
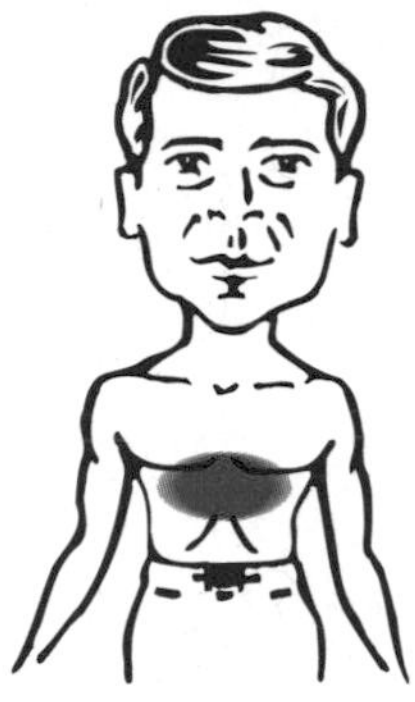

Instead of in the chest, a sensation of aching or weakness may occur in one or both arms, to be confused with arthritis or bursitis; in the neck or jaws, seeming like a toothache; or in the upper abdomen, where it is often mistaken as a symptom of indigestion.

OF A HEART ATTACK

Also possibly present—

- **Shortness of breath**
- **Sweating**
- **Nausea**
- **Sudden weakness**

If any of these symptoms appear, call your doctor immediately or get to the hospital emergency room by the quickest available means.

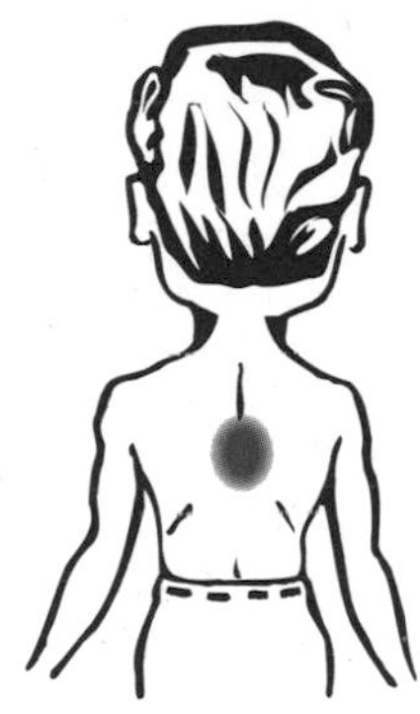

Pain may appear only in the back, commonly between the shoulder blades.

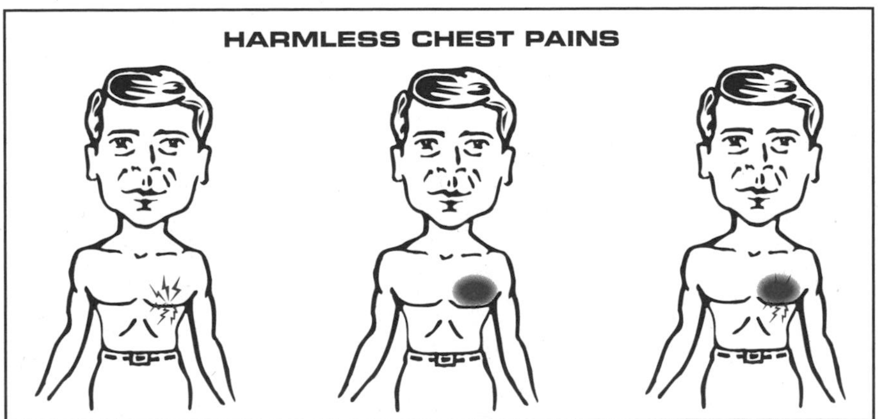

Pain centered near the left nipple is felt by many tense individuals, and is not a sign of a heart attack. This harmless pain is either a sharp jabbing, lasting a second or two, a dull soreness that may persist for hours, or a combination of both. THESE THREE ARE HARMLESS CHEST PAINS.

Notes

Introduction: Why This Book?

1. P. E. Langton and P. L. Thompson, "Helping Heart Attack Victims Save Their Own Lives," *Medical Journal of Australia* (March 3, 1997): 166.

2. According to the American Heart Association, there are 452,300 annual coronary heart disease deaths (mainly from acute myocardial infarction) ("Heart Disease and Stroke Statistics: 2007 Update," *Circulation* [February 6, 2007]: 115, E69–171).

3. According to the *Dictionary of American History*, there were a total of 426,114 U.S. battle deaths in the wars of the twentieth century: 53,402 in World War I; 291,557 in World War II; 33,629 in the Korean War; 47,378 in the Vietnam War; and 148 in the Gulf War (s.v. "Battle Deaths: United States Casualties by Conflict").

4. E. J. Topol, "The Future of Reperfusion," interview by Sylvan Weinberg, *American College of Cardiology Extended Learning* 34, no. 3 (2002).

5. I. Wright et al., "Report of the Committee for the Evaluation of Anticoagulant in Treatment of Coronary Thrombosis with Myocardial Infarction," *American Heart Journal* 36 (1948): 801–15.

6. Glenn O. Turner, "The Missouri Heart Association Early Warning Signs of Heart Attack Public and Professional Education," in *Cardiac Arrest and Resuscitation*, ed. H. E. Stephenson Jr. (St. Louis: C. V. Mosby, 1974), 580–86; Turner, "Speeding Entry into the System: Public Education; The Early Warning Signs," in *The Cardiovascular Care Unit*, ed. Turner (New York: John Wiley and Sons, 1978), 452–53; Turner, "Early Warning Signs of Heart Attack: Three Decades of Public and Professional Education in the Southwest Missouri Ozarks," *Critical Pathways in Cardiology* 2 (2003): 118–24.

Chapter 2. What Is a Heart Attack?

1. P. Rentrop et al., "Reopening of Infarct-Occluded Vessel by Transluminal Recanalisation and Intracoronary Streptokinase Application," *Deutsche Medizin Wochenschrift* 104, no. 41 (1979): 1438–40.

2. Gruppo Italiano per Studie della Streptochinasi Nell'Infarcto Miocardico (GISSI), "Effectiveness of Intravenous Thrombolytic Treatment in Acute Myocardial Infarction," *Lancet* 1 (1986): 397–402.

3. W. D. Weaver et al., "Prehospital-Initiated vs. Hospital-Initiated Thrombolytic Therapy: The Myocardial Infarction Triage and Intervention (MITI) Trial," *Journal of the American Medical Association* 270 (1993): 1211–16.
4. W. D. Weaver, interview by Richard Conti, in *American College of Cardiology Extended Learning Audiotape Series*, ed. Richard Conti (June 2003).

Chapter 3. Heart Attack Early Warning Signs: Your Key to Survival

1. J. G. Canto et al., "Prevalence, Clinical Characteristics, and Mortality among Patients with Myocardial Infarction Presenting without Chest Pain," *Journal of the American Medical Association* 283 (2000): 3223.
2. "Heart Disease and Stroke Statistics: 2007 Update."

Chapter 5. How to Get Proper—and Prompt—Treatment for a Heart Attack

1. R. V. Luepker et al., "Effect of a Community Intervention on Patient Delay and Emergency Medical Service Use in Acute Coronary Heart Disease: The Rapid Early Action for Coronary Treatment (REACT) Trial," *Journal of the American Medical Association* 284 (2000): 60–67.
2. I. C. Gilchrist, "Patient Delay before Treatment in Myocardial Infarction," *British Medical Journal* 1 (1973): 535–37; J. M. Rawles and N. E. Haites, "Patient and General Practitioner Delays in Acute Myocardial Infarction," *British Medical Journal* 296 (1988): 882–84; A. T. Wielgosz et al., "Reasons for Patients' Delay in Response to Symptoms of Acute Myocardial Infarction," *Canadian Medical Association Journal* 139 (1988): 853–57; J. W. Leitch, T. Birbara, and B. Freedman, "Factors Influencing the Time from Onset of Chest Pain to Arrival at Hospital," *Medical Journal of Australia* 150 (1989): 6–10; D. Gray et al., "Impact of Hospital Thrombolysis Policy on Out-of-Hospital Response to Suspected Myocardial Infarction," *Lancet* 341 (1993): 654–57.
3. A. B. Simon, M. Feinleib, and H. K. Thompson Jr., "Components of Delay in the Pre-hospital Phase of Acute Myocardial Infarction," *American Journal of Cardiology* 30 (1972): 476; J. S. Schroeder, I. H. Lamb, and M. Hu, "The Prehospital Course of Patients with Chest Pain: Analysis of the Prodromal, Symptomatic, Decision-Making, Transportation, and Emergency Room Periods," *American Journal of Medicine* 64 (1978): 742; A. A. Alonzo, "The Impact of the Family and Lay Others on Care-Seeking during Life-Threatening Episodes of Suspected Coronary Artery Disease," *Social Science Medicine* 22 (1986): 1297.
4. J. Zapka, B. Estabrook, and J. Gilliland, "Health Care Providers' Perspectives on Patient Delay for Seeking Care for Symptoms of Acute Myocardial Infarction," *Health Education and Behavior* 26, no. 5 (1999): 714–33.
5. Luepker et al., "Community Intervention," 60–67.
6. Turner, "Missouri Heart Association," 580–86; Turner, "Speeding Entry," 452–53; Turner, "Early Warning Signs," 118–24 (for all, see introduction, n. 6).
7. N. Dean, P. Haug, and P. Hawker, "Effect of Mobile Paramedic Units on Outcome in Patients with Myocardial Infarction," *Annals of Emergency Medicine* 17 (1988): 1034–41.
8. L. Becker, M. Larsen, and M. Eisenberg, "Incidence of Cardiac Arrest during Self-Transport for Chest Pain," *Annals of Emergency Medicine* (December 1996): 612–16.

9. D. Faxon and C. Lenfant, "Timing Is Everything: Motivating Patients to Call 9–1–1 at Onset of Acute Myocardial Infarction," *Circulation* 104 (2001): 1210–11.

10. J. L. Brown Jr., "An Eight-Month Evaluation of Prehospital 12-Lead Electrocardiogram Monitoring in Baltimore County," *Maryland Medical Journal Supplement* (1997): 64–66.

11. B. Patterson, director, St. John's Hospital Ambulance Service, interview by the author, Springfield, Mo., November 2004.

12. W. D. Weaver, "Prehospital Reperfusion: Lytics and Triage for Primary PCI," *American College of Cardiology Extended Learning* 34, no. 7 (2002).

13. C. B. Hutchings, N. C. Mann, and M. Daya, "Patients with Chest Pain Calling 9–1–1 or Self-Transporting to Reach Definitive Care: Which Mode Is Quicker?" *American Heart Journal* 147 (2004): 35–41.

14. Becker, "Incidence of Cardiac Arrest," 612–16.

15. J. G. Canto et al., "Use of Emergency Medical Services in Acute Myocardial Infarction and Subsequent Quality of Care," *Circulation* 106 (2002): 3018–23.

16. Ibid.

17. Resource Center, American Hospital Association, Chicago, staff report to author, June 9, 2006.

18. W. W. O'Neal, "Does 90 Minute Door-to-Balloon Time Really Matter in STEMI?" *American College of Cardiology Extended Learning* 37, no. 12 (2005).

19. E. H. Bradley et al., "Strategies for Reducing the Door-to-Balloon Time in Acute Myocardial Infarction," *New England Journal of Medicine* 355, no. 22 (2006): 2308–20.

20. C. L. Grines, "Infarct Angioplasty in the Community. *American College of Cardiology Extended Learning* 36, no. 8 (2004).

Chapter 7. Thrombolysis: The Heart Attack Treatment Breakthrough

1. Rentrop et al., "Infarct-Occluded Vessel," 1438–40 (see chap. 2, n. 1).

2. GISSI, "Intravenous Thrombolytic Treatment," 397–402 (see chap. 2, n. 2).

3. W. D. Weaver, "STEMI: Outcomes with Lysis vs. PCII at >2H, 2–4H, 4–12H," *American College of Cardiology Extended Learning* 35, no. 6 (2003).

4. Weaver et al., "Thrombolytic Therapy," 1211–16 (see chap. 2, n. 3).

5. Third International Study of Infarct Survival Collaborative Group, "ISIS-3: A Randomized Trial of Streptokinase vs. Tissue Plasminogen Activator vs. Anistreplase and of Aspirin Plus Heparin vs. Aspirin Alone among 41,299 Cases of Suspected Acute Myocardial Infarction," *Lancet* 339 (1992): 753–70; GUSTO Investigators, "An International Randomized Trial Comparing Four Thrombolytic Strategies for Acute Myocardial Infarction," *New England Journal of Medicine* 329 (1993): 673–82.

6. P. Chareonthaitawe et al., "The Impact of Time to Thrombolysis Treatment on Outcome in Patients with Acute Myocardial Infarction," *Heart* 84, no. 2 (2000): 142–48.

Chapter 8. Coronary Angiograms: What Are They and What Do They Accomplish?

1. M. Sones, "Coronary Angiography Report," American Heart Association Annual Meeting, General Session, Miami, 1960.

Chapter 9. Balloon Coronary Angioplasty: What It Accomplishes, What It Does Not Accomplish, and How This Affects Your Choices about Treatment

1. A. Gruentzig, "Results from Coronary Angioplasty and Implications for the Future," *American Heart Journal* 103, no. 4 (1982): 779–83.

2. "Heart Disease and Stroke Statistics: 2007 Update."

3. W. E. Boden et al., "Optimal Medical Therapy with or without PCI for Stable Coronary Disease," *New England Journal of Medicine* 356, no. 15 (2007): 1503–16.

4. Ibid.

5. M. Marchione, "Drugs Can Treat Clogged Arteries as Well as Stents," *Associated Press,* March 30, 2007.

6. C. R. Conti, "Restenosis after Angioplasty: Have We Found the Holy Grail?" *American College of Cardiology Extended Learning* 33, no. 12 (2001).

7. C. R. Conti, "Drug-Eluting Stents: Safety Concerns." *American College of Cardiology Extended Learning* 38, no. 11 (2006); Renu Virmani, "Drug-Eluting Stents: Quo Vadis." *American College of Cardiology Extended Learning* 38, no. 12 (2006).

8. American College of Cardiology / American Heart Association Task Force on Practice Guidelines, "ACC / AHA Guidelines for the Management of Patients with ST-Elevation Myocardial Infarction: A Report of the Committee to Revise the 1999 Guidelines for the Management of Patients with Acute Myocardial Infarction," *Journal of the American College of Cardiology* 44, no. 3 (2004): E1-E211.

9. J. W. Kennedy et al., "Recent Changes in Management of Acute Myocardial Infarction: Implications for Emergency Care Physicians," *Journal of the American College of Cardiology* 11, no. 2 (1988): 446–49.

10. American College of Cardiology / American Heart Association Task Force, "ACC / AHA Guidelines," E1-E211.

11. Grines, "Infarct Angioplasty" (see chap. 5, n. 20).

12. S. Borzak, "No Time to Wait," *American Heart Journal* 138 (1999): 1003–4; B. R. Brodie et al., "Importance of Time to Reperfusion for 30-Day and Late Survival Recovery of Left Ventricular Function after Primary Angioplasty for Acute Myocardial Infarction," *Journal of the American College of Cardiology* 32, no. 5 (1998): 1312–19; A. M. Ross, "Remaining Important Problems: Controversies Concerning Reperfusion Therapy for STEMI," *American College of Cardiology Extended Learning* 36, no. 9 (2004).

13. O'Neal, "Door-to-Balloon Time" (see chap. 5, n. 18).

14. E. J. Topol, address at the Mid-America Heart Institute, Kansas City, Mo., 1988.

15. R. J. Gibbons et al., "The Quantification of Infarct Size," *Journal of the American College of Cardiology* 44, no. 8 (2004).

16. E. H. Bradley et al., "Reducing the Door-to-Balloon Time," 2308–20 (see chap. 5, n. 19).

17. B. J. Gersh, "Recorded Remarks, "*American College of Cardiology Extended Learning* 36, no. 10 (2004).

18. C. W. Stone and D. A. Cox, "Recorded Remarks," *American College of Cardiology Extended Learning* 36, no. 10 (2004).

19. P. S. Steg, "Immediate PCI for STEMI: Transport Then Do It?" *American College of Cardiology Extended Learning* 36, no. 8 (2004).

20. T. A. Stukel, F. L. Lucas, and D. E. Wennberg, "Long-Term Outcomes of Regional Variations in Intensity of Invasive vs. Medical Management of

Medicare Patients with Acute Myocardial Infarction," *Journal of the American Medical Association* 293, no. 11 (2005): 1329–37.

21. J. S. Hochman et al., "Coronary Intervention for Persistent Occlusion after Myocardial Infarction," *New England Journal of Medicine* 355 (2006): 2395–2407.

22. C. Scott, reporting for the St. John's Regional Health Center Cardiac Catheterization Laboratory: the charge for a balloon coronary angioplasty, single vessel, with one drug-eluting stent: $17,155 (Springfield, Mo., January 13, 2005); Medicare Web site display of allowances for physician services, Missouri, November 23, 2005: cardiac catheterization, coronary angiography, balloon coronary angioplasty, and stent insertion: $2,619; intravenous administration of thrombolysis agent: $300; Grove Pharmacy, quotation to the author of manufacturers' 2006 charges to hospitals for the two leading thrombolysis drugs: $2,500 and $3,000 (hospitals add markups to these costs in billing patients), Springfield, Mo., 2006.

23. C. R. Conti, "Should Thrombolysis Therapy Be Given to Patients before Urgent PCI?" *American College of Cardiology Extended Learning* 38, no. 3 (2006).

24. Canto et al., "Emergency Medical Services," 3018–23 (see chap. 5, n. 15).

25. R. G. Smalling, unpublished interview by the author, August 2005.

26. S. W. McMurray, unpublished interview by the author, August 2005.

27. D. R. Holmes Jr., B. J. Gersh, and S. G. Ellis, "Rescue Percutaneous Coronary Intervention after Failed Fibrinolytic Therapy: Have Expectations Been Met?" *American Heart Journal* 151 (2006): 779–85.

28. Steg, "Immediate PCI for STEMI."

Chapter 10. Coronary Artery Surgery

1. "Memorial Tribute to Dr. Rene G. Favaloro," *Texas Heart Institute Journal* 31 (2004): 47–60.

2. "Heart Disease and Stroke Statistics: 2007 Update."

Chapter 14. Homocysteine Excess: A New Puzzle

1. K. S. McCully, *The Homocysteine Revolution* (New Canaan, Conn.: Keats Publishing, 1997).

Chapter 15. An Urgent Message: Learn the Early Warning Signs of a Stroke

1. A. T. Schneider et al., "Trends in Community Knowledge of the Warning Signs and Risk Factors for Stroke," *Journal of the American Medical Association* 289 (2003): 343–46.

Chapter 19. Atrial Fibrillation: A Neglected Cause of Strokes

1. American Heart Association, "Heart Disease and Stroke Statistics: 2006 Update," ed. Nancy Haas (Dallas: American Heart Association, 2006).

Chapter 28. What's Wrong with Low-Carb Diets—and What You Should Know about How Much Carbohydrates, Fat, and Protein to Include in Your Diet

1. R. C. Atkins, *The Atkins Diet Revolution* (New York: D. McKay, 1972).
2. R. C. Atkins, *Atkins for Life* (New York: St. Martin's Press, 2003).
3. M. R. Eades and M. D. Eades, *Protein Power* (New York: Bantam Books, 1996).
4. A. Agatston, *The South Beach Diet* (Emmaus, Pa.: Rodale, 2003).
5. F. Pescatore, *The Hamptons Diet* (Hoboken, N.J.: John Wiley and Sons, 2004).
6. R. M. Krauss, "The Effect of Carbohydrate Restriction and Weight Loss on Atherogenic Dyslipidemia," *American College of Cardiology Extended Learning* 36, no. 4 (2004).

Chapter 33. What Is a Proper Exercise Program?

1. K. M. Rexrode et al., "Physical Activity and Coronary Heart Disease in Women: Is 'No Pain, No Gain' Passé?" *Journal of the American Medical Association* 285 (2001): 1447–54.

Chapter 35. Should You Take Weight-Loss Medications?

1. E. M. Guarneri, "Evidence-Based Herbal Medicine—What Works, What Doesn't—Dangerous Interactions," *American College of Cardiology Extended Learning* 36, no. 7 (2004).

Chapter 36. Lifesaving Breakthroughs in Drug Treatment for Cholesterol and Triglycerides

1. C. P. Cannon, "Pravastatin or Atorvastatin Evaluation and Infection Therapy: Thrombolysis in Myocardial Infarction 22 (PROVE IT–TIMI 22)—Statin Comparison," *American College of Cardiology Extended Learning* 36, no. 7 (2004).
2. S. E. Nissen, "REVERSAL: A Prospective, Randomized, Double Blind, Multi-center Study Comparing the Effects of Atorvastatin vs. Pravastatin on the Progression of Coronary Atherosclerotic Lesions as Measured by Intravascular Ultrasound," *American College of Cardiology Extended Learning* 36, no. 3 (2004).
3. S. M. Grundy et al., "Implications of Recent Clinical Trials for the National Cholesterol Education Program Adult Treatment Panel 3 Guidelines," *Circulation* 110 (2004): 227–39.
4. K. von Bergmann, T. Sudhop, and D. Lutjohann, "Cholesterol and Plant Sterol Absorption: Recent Insights" (review), *American Journal of Cardiology* 96, no. 1A (2005): 10D–14D; C. M. Ballantyne et al., "Efficacy and Safety of Ezetimibe Co-administered with Simvastatin Compared with Atorvastatin in Adults with Hypercholesterolemia," *American Journal of Cardiology* 93, no. 12 (2004): 1487–94; Ballantyne et al., "Dose-Comparison Study of the Combination of Ezetimibe and Simvastatin (Vytorin) versus Atorvastatin in Patients with Hypercholesterolemia—the Vytorin versus Atorvastatin (VYVA) Study," *Amer-*

ican Heart Journal 149, no. 3 (2005): 464–73; Ballantyne et al., "Rationale for Targeting Multiple Lipid Pathways for Optimal Cardiovascular Risk Reduction" (review), *American Journal of Cardiology* 96, no. 9A (2005): 14K–19K.

5. J. P. Kastelein et al., "Comparison of Ezetimibe Plus Simvastatin versus Simvastatin Monotherapy on Atherosclerosis Progression in Familial Hypercholesterolemia: Design and Rationale of the Ezetimibe and Simvastatin in Hypercholesterolemia Enhances Atherosclerosis Regression (ENHANCE) Trial," *American Heart Journal* 149 (2005): 234–39.

Chapter 37. Cholesterol and Other Blood Testing: What Tests Should You Have, Where Should You Get Them, and Who Should Administer Them?

1. W. F. Enos, R. H. Holmes, and J. Beyer, "Coronary Disease among United States Soldiers Killed in Action in Korea: Preliminary Report," *Journal of the American Medical Association* 152 (1953): 1090–93.

2. G. S. Berenson et al., "Atherosclerosis of the Aorta and Coronary Arteries and Cardiovascular Risk Factors in Persons Aged 6 to 30 Years and Studied at Necropsy (the Bogalusa Heart Study)," *American Journal of Cardiology* 70 (1992): 851–58.

Chapter 38. Should You Take Aspirin Regularly?

1. V. Fuster, "Tape Recorded Address," *American College of Cardiology Extended Learning* 36, no. 3 (2004).

Chapter 39. Why Smoking Causes Heart Attacks and Strokes—and How I Stopped Smoking

1. R. Doll et al., "Mortality in Relation to Smoking: 40 Years' Observations on Male British Doctors," *British Medical Journal* 309 (1994): 1–11.

Chapter 40. Blood Pressure Control: A Neglected Medical Milestone

1. L. J. Appel, "The Verdict from ALLHAT: Thiazide Diuretics Are the Preferred Initial Therapy for Hypertension," *Journal of the American Medical Association* 288 (2002): 3039.

2. D. Shapiro et al., "Reduction in Drug Requirements for Hypertension by Means of a Cognitive-Behavioral Intervention," *American Journal of Hypertension* 10 (1997): 9–17; P. C. North, "Randomised Controlled Trial of Yoga and Biofeedback in Management of Hypertension," *Lancet,* no. 2 (1975): 93–95; E. Ernst, "Complementary/Alternative Medicine for Hypertension: A Mini-review," *Wien Medizin Wochenschrift* 155 (2005): 386–91.

Chapter 41. What Every Woman Should Know about Coronary Disease in Women

1. American Heart Association, "Heart Disease and Stroke Statistics: 2006 Update."

2. J. E. Manson et al., "A Prospective Study of Obesity and Risk of Coronary Heart Disease in Women," *New England Journal of Medicine* 322, no. 13 (1990): 882–89.

Index

References to illustrations appear in italics.

About the Author

Dr. Glenn O. Turner is a Fellow of the Council on Clinical Cardiology of the American Heart Association and author of *The Cardiovascular Care Unit: A Guide for Planning and Operation.*

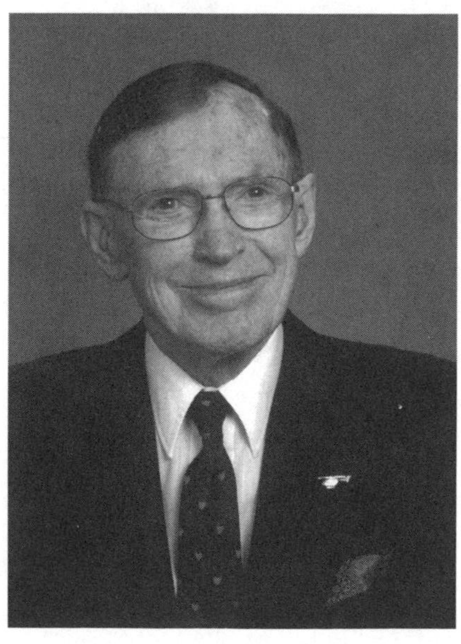

The Missouri Heart Program

Early Warning Signs Wallet/Purse Card

Give a card to your loved ones.

The Early Warning Signs of a Heart Attack

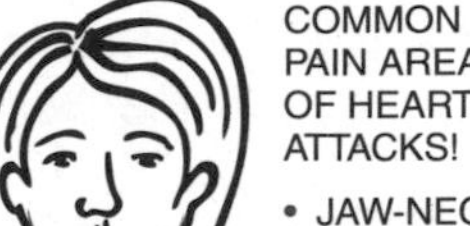

They can come during exercise or rest, day or night.

The Missouri Heart Program

COMMON PAIN AREAS OF HEART ATTACKS!

- JAW-NECK
- CENTER OF FRONT OF CHEST OR BACK
- UPPER ABDOMEN
- ONE OR BOTH ARMS

The Early Warning Signs of a Heart Attack

They can come during exercise or rest, day or night.

The Missouri Heart Program

COMMON PAIN AREAS OF HEART ATTACKS!

- JAW-NECK
- CENTER OF FRONT OF CHEST OR BACK
- UPPER ABDOMEN
- ONE OR BOTH ARMS

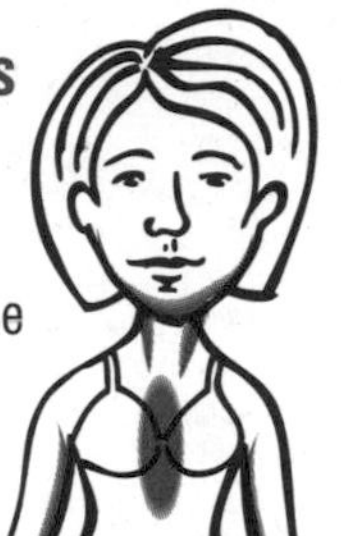

The Early Warning Signs of a Heart Attack

They can come during exercise or rest, day or night.

The Missouri Heart Program

COMMON PAIN AREAS OF HEART ATTACKS!

- JAW-NECK
- CENTER OF FRONT OF CHEST OR BACK
- UPPER ABDOMEN
- ONE OR BOTH ARMS

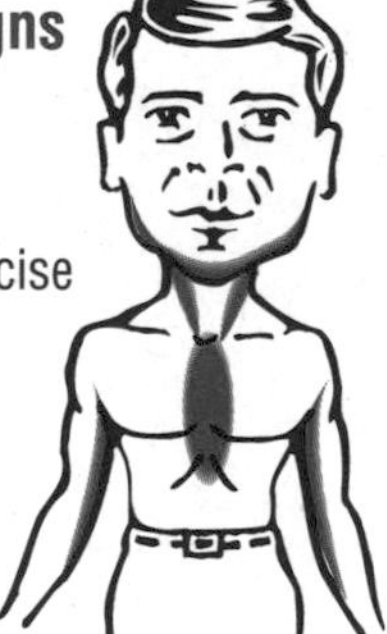

The Early Warning Signs of a Heart Attack

They can come during exercise or rest, day or night.

The Missouri Heart Program

COMMON PAIN AREAS OF HEART ATTACKS!

- JAW-NECK
- CENTER OF FRONT OF CHEST OR BACK
- UPPER ABDOMEN
- ONE OR BOTH ARMS

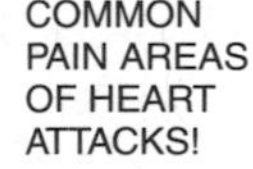

The Early Warning Signs of a Heart Attack

Discomfort in the center of the chest—pressure, fullness, squeezing, aching or burning, possibly extending into one or both arms, the neck, jaws, upper abdomen, or back. It may occur in any one or all these areas without being in the front of the chest. Sweating, shortness of breath, nausea or sudden weakness also may be present. If you experience discomfort in any of these areas,

CALL YOUR DOCTOR!

____

YOUR DOCTOR'S NUMBERS

If your doctor is not immediately available, get to your hospital emergency room by the quickest available means. If you seem severely ill or have no other way to go, **call 9-1-1.**

The Early Warning Signs of a Heart Attack

Discomfort in the center of the chest—pressure, fullness, squeezing, aching or burning, possibly extending into one or both arms, the neck, jaws, upper abdomen, or back. It may occur in any one or all these areas without being in the front of the chest. Sweating, shortness of breath, nausea or sudden weakness also may be present. If you experience discomfort in any of these areas,

CALL YOUR DOCTOR!

____

YOUR DOCTOR'S NUMBERS

If your doctor is not immediately available, get to your hospital emergency room by the quickest available means. If you seem severely ill or have no other way to go, **call 9-1-1.**

The Early Warning Signs of a Heart Attack

Discomfort in the center of the chest—pressure, fullness, squeezing, aching or burning, possibly extending into one or both arms, the neck, jaws, upper abdomen, or back. It may occur in any one or all these areas without being in the front of the chest. Sweating, shortness of breath, nausea or sudden weakness also may be present. If you experience discomfort in any of these areas,

CALL YOUR DOCTOR!

____

YOUR DOCTOR'S NUMBERS

If your doctor is not immediately available, get to your hospital emergency room by the quickest available means. If you seem severely ill or have no other way to go, **call 9-1-1.**

The Early Warning Signs of a Heart Attack

Discomfort in the center of the chest—pressure, fullness, squeezing, aching or burning, possibly extending into one or both arms, the neck, jaws, upper abdomen, or back. It may occur in any one or all these areas without being in the front of the chest. Sweating, shortness of breath, nausea or sudden weakness also may be present. If you experience discomfort in any of these areas,

CALL YOUR DOCTOR!

____

YOUR DOCTOR'S NUMBERS

If your doctor is not immediately available, get to your hospital emergency room by the quickest available means. If you seem severely ill or have no other way to go, **call 9-1-1.**

The Missouri Heart Program

Early Warning Signs Wallet/Purse Card

Give a card to your loved ones.